WORKBOOK FOR COGNITIVE SKILLS

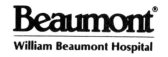
William Beaumont Hospital

*A complete listing of the books in this series
can be found online at wsupress.wayne.edu*

Series Editors
Michael I. Rolnick, Ph.D., CCC-SLP
William Beaumont Hospital

Alex Johnson, Ph.D., CCC-SLP
MGH Institute of Health Professions

WORKBOOK FOR COGNITIVE SKILLS

Exercises for Thought Processing and Word Retrieval

Second Edition
Revised and Updated

Susan Howell Brubaker, M.S., CCC-SLP

Wayne State University Press
Detroit

ISBN: 978-0-8143-3313-6

First edition © 1987 by Wayne State University Press.

∞ The paper used in this publication meets the minimum requirements of the
American National Standard for Information Sciences—Permanence of Paper
for Printed Library Materials, ANSI Z39.48-1984.

CONTENTS

ABOUT THE AUTHOR

For more than thirty years, Susan Howell Brubaker has worked in the Speech and Language Pathology Department at William Beaumont Hospital, Royal Oak, Michigan. She has specialized in working with adults who have suffered communicative loss as a result of neurological dysfunction or brain injury. She holds the B.S. from St. Lawrence University, Canton, New York, the M.S. from Ithaca College, Ithaca, New York, and the Certificate of Clinical Competence from the American Speech-Language-Hearing Association.

Other Susan Howell Brubaker books published by Wayne State University Press:

Sourcebook for Receptive and Expressive Language Functioning

Basic Level Workbook for Aphasia

Workbook for Aphasia:
Exercises for Expressive and Receptive Language Functioning

Workbook for Language Skills:
Exercises for Written and Verbal Expression

Workbook for Reasoning Skills:
Exercises for Functional Reasoning and Reading Comprehension

Clinicians working with individuals having language and cognitive impairments are constantly in search of appropriate and interesting treatment materials. The Brubaker workbooks have become *the* professional standards and best sellers since their inception and with good reason. These publications are designed by a master clinician who has the ability and fortitude to create and, lucky for us, share her ideas. When a new Brubaker book is published, one is drawn to its theme and its contents, for in it is Susan Howell Brubaker's latest contribution to the rehabilitation of persons with language and cognitive dysfunction.

The *Workbook for Cognitive Skills* (the red book) stands out from other materials. It presents a richness in the variety of clinical activities and a multiplicity of formats for the user. Every attempt is made to use extensive vocabulary and to provide maximum language stimulation. Special emphasis is given to word retrieval and the development of problem-solving strategies. Functionality, use of everyday and cultural terms, names, and titles make this workbook relevant and timely for both adolescents and older adults.

Of special interest is the CLUES section provided in the yellow-tabbed section. The unique CLUES concept allows users tremendous flexibility and help in completing the pages. It provides examples of useful strategies to help work through an exercise and allows those who do not have spelling or writing skills to also use the book. While some patients will only require the CLUES section to help with one or two questions, others can use it for the multiple-choice answers or for checking their work. The CLUES section adds another dimension to the patient's treatment, for it becomes part of the therapeutic process to locate correct answers from among those listed.

Finally, the exercises included in this book are not only novel and challenging, but they are also fun. The rehabilitation process can be frustrating and grueling. Susan Howell Brubaker has recognized the value of humor and variety during recovery. Many of the puzzles and exercises provide a welcome smile along with a challenge while aiding in treatment. We provide our patients with their own book as we have found they enjoy carrying it and working through exercises whether or not they are assigned.

This revised and updated version keeps the most popular tasks and adds new challenges that use current references. Welcome to the newest version of the Brubaker series of exceptionally solid and widely applicable clinical tools.

Michael I. Rolnick, Ph.D., CCC-SLP, Director
Speech and Language Pathology Department
William Beaumont Hospital
Royal Oak, Michigan

INTRODUCTION

As we improve and revise the Brubaker workbook series, we look to the users—patients and professionals—to give us feedback. We have listened and field-tested this edition so it is even better and more versatile than its previous best-selling version.

What's new on the outside?

- A new ring binder that retains the familiar and sturdy cover with the name on the spine so it can be easily identified on a shelf

- Separate sheets of paper that are easily removed so you can take out just one or two exercises

- Heavier paper that is durable but not too heavy to put through a normal copier

- Tabbed dividers to help you locate exercises more quickly and easily

- Large bold print on the dividers to make it easy to flip to the target area of your choice

What's new on the inside?

- Pages that have a new look with clean lines and good visual divisions

- Rewritten directions that are direct and to-the-point

- New and revised exercises—some that were made more challenging and some that were clarified or tweaked to add interest

- Larger and easier-to-read print with more horizontal lines between questions to help those with visual difficulties

- Examples used more judiciously to add to the challenge, for problem-solving, and for new learning

- Larger and bolder page numbers

- Additional margin space, space within and between questions, and improved spacing in the writing areas

- More than 70 pages of entirely new exercises

- More than 1,000 questions revised to be more contemporary and engaging

- More complete and usable *CLUES* section

- Better-placed exercises in target areas that reflect their focus

- Two user's guides—one for the exercises and one for the CLUES—added to give instructions and helpful suggestions

- Suggestions for Strategies added to assist users in working through the exercises added in the CLUES section

- Assignments page added to help users keep track of what has to be done and provide a useful record of progress over time

- Revised copyright statement that grants you permission to legally copy exercises for your personal use or for that of a patient

We believe we have encompassed the best of your ideas and the best of the original book that has become so popular. We hope you agree that this revised and updated edition is a much-improved tool to help you the user or you the clinician achieve your goals.

Thank you for your continued support of Brubaker books, your feedback, and your dedication to using our treatment materials to stimulate the brain, provide practice, a challenge, and perhaps even a chuckle or two.

This version of *Workbook for Cognitive Skills* is extremely versatile because of the addition of the CLUES section. This unique concept makes the book appropriate for patients at varying levels of function. It also eliminates the need for good spelling skills as the patient can copy words for the answers. The CLUES section offers the first answer, hints to the answer, part of the answer, or the answers in scrambled or alphabetical order. Read more about this tool in the Introduction to the CLUES Section on the next page.

The book is divided into six different target areas with 111 exercises of varying length and complexity. The exercises can be completed in any order. Some are easier and some are more difficult, but which is which depends on the individuals working with the book, their particular strengths, and what would be challenging to them.

Below are some suggestions to maximize the usefulness and functionality of the workbook.

- Rather than explaining the directions for each task, allow users to read the directions as a way to further call on their cognitive skills. The completed example was deliberately left out of this edition to require the patient to use the written directives.

- As a functional way of improving auditory comprehension and retention, provide a verbal explanation for each exercise, then require the patient to restate the explanation.

- Give your patients a personal copy of this workbook during their rehabilitation to enhance their ability to follow through with treatment tasks and for carryover. At our facility, we identify exercises that reinforce the goal addressed in treatment and assign them

for completion prior to the next session. These assignments can be written on the assignments sheet on page 15. You can also reinforce strategies you are working on by marking them on the list of strategies on page 13.

- The use of this workbook as a home program increases self-direction and initiation, reinforces a sense of accomplishment, confidence, and motivation for greater independence with communication skills. It also frees up time in the treatment session to work on other functional goals that are not conducive to a workbook format.

- Encourage your patients to use the CLUES to correct their own responses and figure out the reasons for the discrepancies between answers. They can also make a case for the accuracy of their own answers. It should be considered that some items have a number of reasonable answers where others must be answered in a certain way according to the directions.

- Having patients note the date and the start and completion time of an exercise can help them monitor their processing time, which helps with building the self-monitoring skills necessary for managing impulsiveness and improving speed of processing. The date is helpful as a reference to remind patients of their improvements and work.

- The added value of this book is that in order to get through many of the exercises, patients have to use reasoning and problem-solving skills to deduce possible answers, figure out a next step, or even work backward. This makes it more than just a language or word-finding task.

- The inclusion of families and caregivers is paramount in a successful recovery. In our facility, families and caregivers take an active role in the rehabilitation process. They observe and participate in the use of this workbook. We instruct the caregiver on when and how to help as well as how not to help. We usually assign pages that we feel the patient can handle independently, and then we rely on feedback from the caregiver as to how the patient was or was not able to complete the pages and about other factors such as the time it took, the frustration level, pacing, success, and interest.

We hope these suggestions will be helpful to your caseload and will serve as a catalyst for your own ideas.

Lisa M. Mammoser, M.A., CCC-SLP
Coordinator, Diagnostics Program
Center for Adult Communication Disorders
Speech and Language Pathology Department

Carolyn A. Doty, M.A., CCC-SLP
Manager, Adult Outpatient Services
Center for Adult Communication Disorders
Speech and Language Pathology Department

William Beaumont Hospital
Royal Oak, Michigan

USER'S GUIDE TO THE <u>CLUES</u> SECTION (YELLOW TAB)

The final yellow-tabbed section marked CLUES is a unique and important addition to this book. The CLUES section was conceived as a way to help individuals with limited spelling, writing, word-finding, and/or reasoning skills complete the exercises. It has done that, and it has also added an extra dimension to the book.

The added tasks of locating the page the user needs, figuring out the type of CLUES that are given, and actually going between the exercise and the CLUES are challenging in their own right but for different reasons than the skills needed in the original exercise.

We have seen professionals who give the task purely for the purpose of finding the answers from CLUES and putting them where they should go. An even more creative use is to assign a range of pages and provide a list of random answers from CLUES. The patient has to discover and list what page and what question the answer comes from.

The CLUES section can be used in the following ways:

1. To learn strategies that will help users when working an exercise
2. To provide non-spellers with means to copy answers from a scrambled format into their correct placement in an exercise
3. To provide users who could not use the book without CLUES expanded options to complete the exercises with a feeling of accomplishment
4. To provide just a clue, a hint, a partial answer, or just one answer to help users complete a question or understand a concept
5. To serve as a modified version of an Answer Key
6. To provide users with suggestions and types of strategies to help them as they work

through the book and its wide variety of exercises

The next page lists a number of strategies that users can employ to help them approach the exercises or if they get stuck. There is a check box next to each one so that the best strategies for that user can be marked.

The CLUES section lists exercises by page number. Each exercise will show a set of clues most appropriate for that exercise. In many cases, the clue is a scrambled or alphabetized list of answers, but it could also be part of an answer (e.g., the first two letters), hints about how to approach the problem, or another type of clue.

The only exercises not included in CLUES are those that already have multiple-choice answers within the exercise. The Strategies list has suggestions for how to approach these pages.

If a patient is having difficulty with flipping back-and-forth between the CLUES section and the page being worked on, take the CLUES page out of the binder (or photocopy it) and put it next to the page being worked on.

In some cases, the use of CLUES should be discouraged other than to check answers after the individuals have completed an exercise. Users can become overly reliant on digging out answers rather than attempting to figure it out on their own.

And finally, for the professional, CLUES does serve as a modified answer key. Many of the exercises can be checked as they are read through—the answer either fits or makes sense or it does not. Consider alternate answers as an opportunity to have patients explain their thinking. The insight you gain from that may be valuable clinical information.

STRATEGIES AND SUGGESTIONS FOR COMPLETING THE EXERCISES

This section lists some strategies and suggestions to help you work through the exercises. Read through them before you start an exercise or if you get stuck. The box next to each suggestion is provided so you can check the strategies that will be most helpful to you.

☐ Read through the entire directions and make sure you understand them before starting.

☐ Use a pencil with a big, soft eraser.

☐ If you have exercises with a list of answer choices, cross out each answer as you use it.

☐ Fill in all the answers you know, then go back and start the harder ones.

☐ When you have a list of possible answers, try each one in order to see what might fit. Go in order when you try the choices—the usual way is top to bottom or left to right. Don't skip around or you will lose track of what you have already tried.

☐ When you have a list of answer choices, go through the list and eliminate any choices you know are wrong by lightly marking "X" next to them. If you do not find the answer, you can go through the choices again and only look at the choices that you did NOT cross out.

☐ Erase your pencil marks when you find an answer so you can start over with the next question.

☐ When you have two columns to match an answer, use the left column as the anchor column. Start with the first question and try each choice from the right column in order until you find the answer. Do the same with the second question.

☐ Use the alphabet for exercises when you need to insert letters or think of words. The alphabet is written at the top of pages 123, 124, and 125. You could copy it to another sheet and keep it next to the page on which you are working. Try the letters in order in the word. Lightly write a possible letter so you can visualize if a word looks right, then erase it if it is wrong. Go to the next letter and repeat the process. When you get the correct letter(s), write it darker and erase your other marks.

☐ When you go through the alphabet to find letters in a word, try one letter in all the blanks of all the words. When you find where that letter goes, try the next letter. If the letter can be used more than once, write it lightly next to all the words in which it can go.

☐ When you are inserting letters in a word, consider how the word looks. Some letter combinations don't work, and in some places it is obvious that a vowel is missing.

☐ When a letter(s) is missing in a word, look at it and see if you can visualize the whole word.

☐ If you are filling in letters, write the word and the blanks on another sheet of paper so you can see it by itself. This can help you visualize a word.

☐ Say the word or phrase out loud. Look away from the page and say it. Listen to the sound.

☐ When the exercise gives words in categories, take a sheet of paper and write some words in that category. Then go back to the page and see if any of them fit.

☐ In crossword grids, look at the length of words as well as the order of letters and where they would cross. Write in the longest or shortest words first.

☐ In word searches, find the first letter of the word you are looking for. From that letter, look in all directions to see if the other letters of the word are there.

☐ If a blank line represents a word, read the phrase out loud and use "um" or the word "blank" for the missing word. Look up from the page and listen to the sound.

☐ If you don't understand how to do an exercise, go to its page in CLUES. This will at least give you the first answer to get you started.

☐ Set up Scrabble or letter tiles that look like the partial words in which letters are missing. Try other letter tiles where the missing letter(s) should be.

☐ Use a blank white sheet of paper to cover up parts of the page so you can see and concentrate on only one question at a time.

☐ For a page with a grid, pictures, maps, calendars, etc., use some sort of order to scan them—from top to bottom or left to right. Do this each time you need to refer to them for an answer.

☐ Lightly make a check in the left margin by questions that you skip over. Then when you return to them, you only need to look at the questions you checked.

☐ If you are stuck, try reading the information slowly and out loud.

☐ If you are really stuck, leave the answer blank and move on. Come back to the question later.

☐ Or if you are really stuck, look up the page in the CLUES section for help.

☐ If you are getting frustrated, put the book down and come back another time.

☐ Take the page you need from the CLUES section out of the binder and put it next to the exercise you are working on.

☐ There will likely be some questions you will not know. You may also think of a different but reasonable answer from what is in CLUES. In addition to challenging your brain, the book is supposed to be fun. Don't let a question or exercise upset you—just skip it and go on or put the book down and return later.

ASSIGNMENTS

Refer to this page to remind you of what you have been assigned to do.

Date Assigned	Date Due	Pages

TARGET AREA 1:
Word Formation

TARGET AREA 1: Word Formation

DIRECTIONS: Write the same letter on all four lines to make words. See **CLUES** for help.

1. ___ and	4. ___ ugs	7. ___ ill
f ___ ag	a ___ le	s ___ ot
ca ___ m	ba ___ y	ca ___ e
tel ___	slo ___	hel ___
2. ___ ice	5. ___ ach	8. ___ ble
s ___ ash	b ___ st	p ___ st
bu ___ p	ov ___ r	cl ___ m
roo ___	wav ___	are ___
3. ___ now	6. ___ ark	9. ___ ust
o ___ ay	i ___ ea	f ___ og
jo ___ e	ti ___ e	wi ___ e
hoo ___	loa ___	bea ___

TARGET AREA 1: Word Formation

*DIRECTIONS: Write the two letters from the gray box that, when added to the letters, will make four different words. See **CLUES** for help.*

am	op	ea	th	st	ce

1. ___ ___ dar

    s ___ ___ ne

    ni ___ ___ r

    dan ___ ___

4. ___ ___ eer

    du ___ ___ y

    wa ___ ___ e

    coa ___ ___

2. ___ ___ ing

    o ___ ___ er

    pa ___ ___ s

    boo ___ ___

5. ___ ___ ger

    w ___ ___ ve

    ch ___ ___ p

    Kor ___ ___

3. ___ ___ use

    c ___ ___ el

    fl ___ ___ e

    cre ___ ___

6. ___ ___ ens

    g ___ ___ her

    sc ___ ___ e

    tro ___ ___

TARGET AREA 1: **Word Formation**

*DIRECTIONS: Write the three letters from the gray box that, when added to the letters, will make four different words. See **CLUES** for help.*

per	ast	eve	gen	ant	tar

1. __ __ __ hem

   w __ __ __ ed

   pl __ __ __ s

   inf __ __ __

2. __ __ __ iod

   o __ __ __ as

   ex __ __ __ t

   dia __ __ __

3. __ __ __ tle

   a __ __ __ cy

   ur __ __ __ t

   oxy __ __ __

4. __ __ __ hma

   c __ __ __ le

   ro __ __ __ s

   bre __ __ __

5. __ __ __ nts

   r __ __ __ al

   el __ __ __ n

   sle __ __ __

6. __ __ __ get

   s __ __ __ ch

   ro __ __ __ y

   gui __ __ __

TARGET AREA 1: Word Formation

Shared Letters

DIRECTIONS: *The three words across each line are missing the same letter. Write that letter at the end of the line. If you choose the correct letter, the name of a flower will read down. See* **CLUES** *for help.*

1. ___ i m   F r e ___   c o ___ e   ___

    s c ___ l d   h ___ v e   g l ___ d   ___

    w a ___ t   ___ t c h   b ___ t e   ___

    t a ___ t e   ___ o l v e   ___ q u e a k   ___

    ___ e s   b u s ___   s p ___   ___

---

2. s h o ___ t   w ___ i n k l e   s h i v e ___   ___

    b ___ n e   f ___ r k   ___ n e   ___

    c o a ___ t   w h i ___ p e r   ___ w i m   ___

    p o c k ___ t   w ___ s t   o v ___ r   ___

---

3. a c ___ i o n   ___ h u n d e r   h a t c h e ___   ___

    r ___ i n   s c r ___ b   ___ n i v e r s e   ___

    ___ a n t e r n   c e l ___ o   g ___ o v e   ___

    i n v a l ___ d   p r ___ n t   s ___ r e n   ___

    s l e e ___ i n g   ___ e a c e   o ___ i n i o n   ___

4. ___ oison   li ___ stick   mum ___ s   _____

   ___ rrow   y ___ rd   exch ___ nge   _____

   mo ___ ey   pea ___ ut   ___ oise   _____

   mi ___ take   pha ___ e   ___ trike   _____

   enjo ___   dizz ___   c ___ clone   _____

5. ___ isitor   ad ___ ice   na ___ y   _____

   mus ___ c   pol ___ cy   shr ___ mp   _____

   ker ___ sene   th ___ rn   ___ lder   _____

   ba ___ d   missi ___ e   At ___ antic   _____

   twic ___   ___ gg   j ___ rk   _____

   ___ rust   jacke ___   pa ___ rol   _____

6. ex ___ ited   ___ onquer   sele ___ tion   _____

   to ___ pedo   bu ___ eau   familia ___   _____

   pers ___ n   b ___ unce   envel ___ pe   _____

   fa ___ e   ___ rystal   s ___ rape   _____

   p ___ ddle   g ___ ilty   j ___ nior   _____

   ma ___ ter   ___ kating   u ___ her   _____

TARGET AREA 1: Word Formation

DIRECTIONS: Combine a word from each column to form a phrase. Write the phrase on the line. The answers on this page are famous people. See **CLUES** *for help.*

1.	James	Allan	Clinton
2.	Kareem	Luther	Carver
3.	George	Earl	Laurent
4.	Yves	Saint	Jones
5.	Martin	Lloyd	King
6.	Hillary	Washington	Wright
7.	Frank	Abdul	Poe
8.	Edgar	Rodham	Jabbar

1. _____

2. _____

3. _____

4. _____

5. _____

6. _____

7. _____

8. _____

Continue as before, but match the three-word food items.

9.	chicken	pea	pie
10.	oatmeal	chow	hash
11.	key	ice	soup
12.	angel	raisin	bread
13.	split	beef	cookie
14.	corned	food	mein
15.	vanilla	cream	sandwich
16.	tuna	nut	cake
17.	ice	lime	sundae
18.	banana	salad	cream

9. _____

10. _____

11. _____

12. _____

13. _____

14. _____

15. _____

16. _____

17. _____

18. _____

Continue as before, but match the three-word titles of TV shows.

19.	Wheel	and	Right
20.	The	My	Raymond
21.	Meet	Loves	Order
22.	I	O'Reilly	Press
23.	Law	of	Children
24.	Saturday	is	America
25.	Everybody	Night	Lucy
26.	Price	Morning	Fortune
27.	All	the	Factor
28.	Good	Love	Live

19. _____

20. _____

21. _____

22. _____

23. _____

24. _____

25. _____

26. _____

27. _____

28. _____

TARGET AREA 1: Word Formation   Word Completion

*DIRECTIONS: Complete each word by adding a letter so that a man or woman's name will form reading down in each column. See **CLUES** for help.*

1. arm ___ est

   rem ___ del

   dri ___ ble

   car ___ ful

   dep ___ ive

   men ___ ion

2. o ___ ey

   l ___ rk

   i ___ is

   a ___ le

3. ___ aw

   ___ re

   ___ ud

   ___ ye

   ___ ki

4. nu ___ get

   sl ___ epy

   ch ___ ose

   pa ___ rot

   bi ___ ger

   sn ___ eze

5. en ___ oy

   st ___ am

   tr ___ in

   pa ___ el

6. fi ___

   ac ___

   fo ___

   he ___

   tr ___

7. e ___ ect

   h ___ aven

   u ___ fair

   a ___ other

   s ___ ngle

   a ___ fection

   r ___ verse

   t ___ affic

10. someti ___ e

   pan ___ c

   tea ___ h

   nig ___ t

   oft ___ n

   footba ___ l

   pil ___ s

   answ ___ r

8. i ___ y

   w ___ s

   a ___ t

   f ___ g

   e ___ k

   r ___ e

   e ___ d

11. ha ___ k

   sk ___ d

   ki ___ l

   wi ___ t

   sh ___ n

   th ___ w

   la ___ b

9. ___ ell

   ___ sual

   ___ cho

12. ___ ime

   int ___ mate

   ti ___ id

TARGET AREA 1: Word Formation

DIRECTIONS: Match a word on the left with a word on the right to form a longer word.
*Write the word on the line. See **CLUES** for help.*

1. ant   ace   _____

   pat   ate   _____

   err   ron   _____

   pal   and   _____

   ash   ore   _____

   men   hem   _____

2. off   son   _____

   bud   ate   _____

   rot   ice   _____

   but   gin   _____

   sea   her   _____

   mar   get   _____

   arc   ton   _____

30

3. char   able   _____

   stub   tone   _____

   plea   coal   _____

   ours   elves   _____

   mono   rain   _____

   reap   rate   _____

   mode   born   _____

   port   sure   _____

   rest   pear   _____

4. shed   tick   _____

   auto   tone   _____

   gems   sing   _____

   brow   rate   _____

   feat   acre   _____

   lips   hers   _____

   must   ding   _____

   gene   ache   _____

   mass   mate   _____

TARGET AREA 1: Word Formation

DIRECTIONS: *Match a letter group on the left with a group on the right to form a word.*
Write the word on the line. See **CLUES** *for help.*

1. emp   oon   _____

   twe   vel   _____

   gra   ire   _____

   obt   rve   _____

   bab   nty   _____

   inc   ain   _____

   sta   ome   _____

2. hyb   uid   _____

   cha   ard   _____

   nor   mal   _____

   abo   pel   _____

   bou   rid   _____

   liq   nce   _____

   sal   ary   _____

3. fami elor   _____

 laug ious   _____

 bach ical   _____

 phys bble   _____

 juve odil   _____

 squa nile   _____

 daff hing   _____

 mack liar   _____

 prev erel   _____

4. roma gany   _____

 humi hful   _____

 acti kade   _____

 trut dity   _____

 bloc ntic   _____

 para ines   _____

 maho dise   _____

 abso vity   _____

 rout lute   _____

TARGET AREA 1: Word Formation

*DIRECTIONS: Choose a word from the right that will fit into the letters on the left to form a word. The order of the letters stays the same. Write the word on the line to show the completed word. See **CLUES** for help.*

1. po _____ ive   rat

    d _____ er   tub

    g _____ eful   sit

    vo _____ ulary   raw

    s _____ born   cab

    pa _____ nt   tie

---

2. p _____ lem   met

    s _____ poo   our

    bu _____ ess   run

    si _____ alk   rob

    te _____ ram   sin

    c _____ ch   dew

    so _____ hing   ham

    res _____ ce   leg

3. e _____ lish   line

   ad _____ ure   rest

   lone _____ ss   lamb

   re _____ nt   stab

   ca _____ ar   side

   w _____ le   reed

   f _____ om   vent

   f _____ oyant   lend

---

4. gui _____ nes   side

   c _____ ed   dust

   s _____ er   hear

   re _____ sal   deli

   nutc _____ er   hang

   in _____ ry   rack

   or _____ nt   ring

   me _____ ue   moth

   pre _____ nt   name

TARGET AREA 1: Word Formation

DIRECTIONS: Choose a word from the right that will fit into the letters on the left so a word is formed. The order of the letters stays the same. Write the letters in order on the blanks. See **CLUES** *for help.*

1. s ___ l ___ n ___   out

    ___ r ___ n ___   nod

    u ___ f ___ l ___   pit

    p ___ r ___ u ___   mud

    ___ o ___ n ___   use

    l ___ c ___ s ___   wig

---

2. ___ c ___ n ___   pub

    ___ h ___ s ___   cut

    ___ l ___ m ___   can

    ___ h ___ i ___   set

    ___ r ___ a ___   bed

    ___ o ___ n ___   got

3. i ___ l ___ n ___   sad

   ___ o ___ r ___ e   pep

   ___ r ___ v ___   pie

   ___ r ___ a ___ h   has

   s ___ r ___ n ___   art

   u ___ k ___ e ___   gay

   p ___ r ___ o ___   tog

   s ___ l ___ c ___   bet

---

4. ___ r ___ m ___ l ___   pose

   ___ e ___ k ___ n ___   tape

   u ___ h ___ l ___ t ___ r   spot

   ___ u ___ p ___ r ___   main

   ___ r ___ t ___ c ___   weed

   ___ o ___ k ___ u ___   poet

   i ___ p ___ t ___ e ___ t   shoe

   ___ c ___ o ___ n ___ r   loot

TARGET AREA 1: Word Formation   Embedded Words

*DIRECTIONS: Each line contains a longer word in which two smaller words are embedded. Pick two short words from the list to fill in the blanks to make the longer word. Each word is used once. See **CLUES** for help.*

1. s ___ ___ ___ p ___ ___ ___   do   and

   c ___ ___ ___ l e h ___ ___ ___ er   no   now

   ___ ___ o r ___ ___ l l   be   oar

   k ___ ___ w l ___ ___ ___ ___   up   low

   t ___ ___ ___ i ___ ___ ___ ___ y   rag   old

   c ___ ___ b ___ ___ ___ d   call   edge

---

2. h ___ ___ b ___ ___ ___ ___ r   am   lot

   p ___ ___ ___ o ___ ___ ___ y   ask   cop

   s ___ ___ ___ e c ___ ___ ___   hot   car

   c ___ ___ ___ h e s ___ ___ ___   read   pin

   b ___ ___ ___ ___ b ___ ___ ___ e t   row   urge

   w ___ ___ ___ f ___ ___ ___ er   all   low

3.   __ __ __ a __ __ __ __ o   arm   her

     __ __ __ __ __ n d __ __ __ t   men   sat

     __ __ __ i s __ __ __ __ i o n   hoe   wit

     s __ __ __ s t __ __ __ __   met   raw

     __ __ __ h d __ __ __ n   ring   fact

     t __ __ __ m o __ __ __ e r   comma   dill

---

4. fel __ __ __ s __ __ __   us   bar

     s __ __ __ n __ __ __ n   hip   city

     __ __ __ __ c i __ __ __ c e   eve   tee

     __ __ __ t __ __ __ e r   coin   den

     h __ __ __ b r __ __ h   pub   air

     __ __ __ l i __ __ __ __   end   low

---

5. in __ __ __ __ i __ __ __ __   hut   at

     __ __ __ h a t __ __ __   art   gate

     __ __ __ a c __ __ __ e   comb   sign

     r e __ __ __ __ a t i __ __   Man   tan

     e __ __ __ h w __ __ m   on   or

     __ __ __ __ i n __ __ i o n   vest   par

TARGET AREA 1: Word Formation

DIRECTIONS: On each line a common word can be created by saying the letter out loud and adding the short word to make a longer word. Write that word on the line. See **CLUES** for help.

1. S + court   _____

2. R + me   _____

3. B + leave   _____

4. C + son   _____

5. A + bull   _____

6. M + ocean   _____

7. B + gun   _____

8. X + plane   _____

9. P + pull   _____

10. L + swear   _____

11. D + bait   _____

12. I + site   _____

13. O + bay   _____

14. R + tickle   _____

15. N + gin   _____

16. blew + J   _____

17. hair + M   _____

18. seed + R   _____

19. air + S   _____

20. crow + K   _____

21. lay + Z   _____

22. fan + C   _____

23. dew + T   _____

24. prayer + E   _____

25. air + 0   _____

26. bran + D   _____

27. gal + N   _____

28. bay + B   _____

29. hey + Z   _____

30. few + L   _____

TARGET AREA 1: Word Formation   Piggyback Words

DIRECTIONS: Write a different word on each line so two compound words (or two-word phrases) are formed. The first compound ends with the word printed, and the second one begins with that word. There are several possible answers. See **CLUES** *for help.*

1. _____ book   book _____

2. _____ side   side _____

3. _____ eye   eye _____

4. _____ man   man _____

5. _____ stand   stand _____

6. _____ be   be _____

7 _____ over   over _____

8. _____ day   day _____

9. _____ sand   sand _____

10. _____ house   house _____

11. _____ down   down _____

12. _____ night   night _____

13. _____ dog   dog _____

14. _____ paper   paper _____

15. _____ bed   bed _____

16. _____ out   out _____

17. _____ town   town _____

18. _____ off   off _____

19. _____ chair   chair _____

20. _____ pan   pan _____

21. _____ hand   hand _____

22. _____ check   check _____

23. _____ play   play _____

24. _____ foot   foot _____

25. _____ work   work _____

TARGET AREA 1: Word Formation   Compound Words

DIRECTIONS: Form several compound words using the word shown as a base. On this page, you will add the last word, and on the next page add the first word of the phrase. There are many possible answers. See **CLUES** *for help.*

1. head _____

   head _____

   head _____

   head _____

   head _____

   head _____

3. back _____

   back _____

   back _____

   back _____

   back _____

   back _____

2. blue _____

   blue _____

   blue _____

   blue _____

   blue _____

   blue _____

4. sun _____

   sun _____

   sun _____

   sun _____

   sun _____

   sun _____

44

5. _____ board

_____ board

_____ board

_____ board

_____ board

_____ board

7. _____ ball

_____ ball

_____ ball

_____ ball

_____ ball

_____ ball

6. _____ light

_____ light

_____ light

_____ light

_____ light

_____ light

8. _____ room

_____ room

_____ room

_____ room

_____ room

_____ room

TARGET AREA 1: Word Formation

Letter Addition

*DIRECTIONS: These puzzles only read across. Drop down any letters you can to the next line and add a new last letter to form a word. Continue until you run out of boxes. There are many possible answers. See **CLUES** for help.*

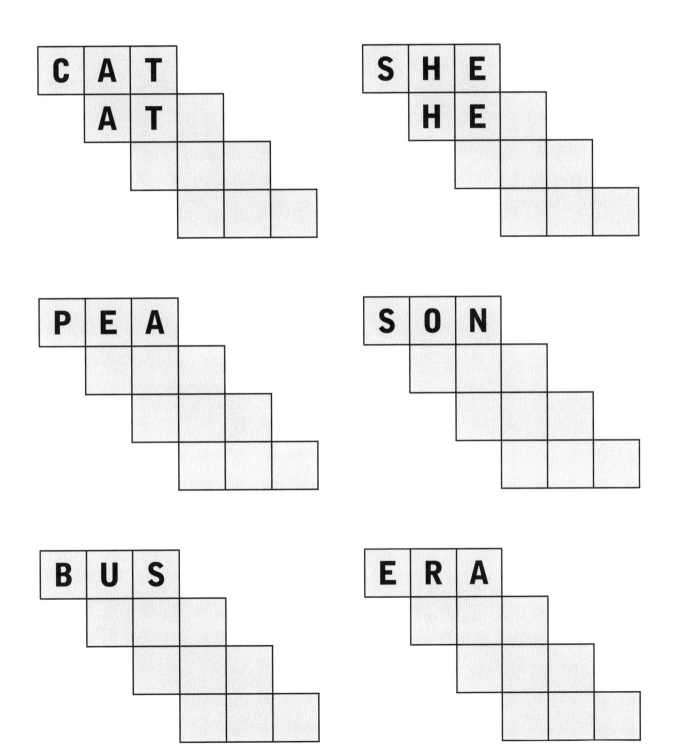

TARGET AREA 1: Word Formation

Category Crosswords

*DIRECTIONS: The crossword grid is partially filled with letters. Add more letters to make the
names of colors reading across and down. See **CLUES** for help.*

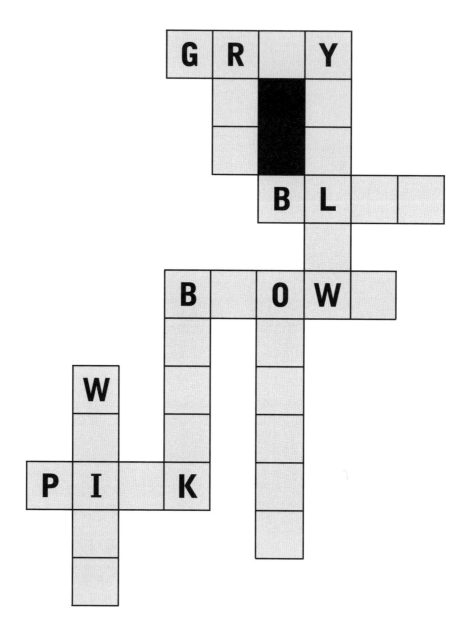

Fill in the names of beverages.

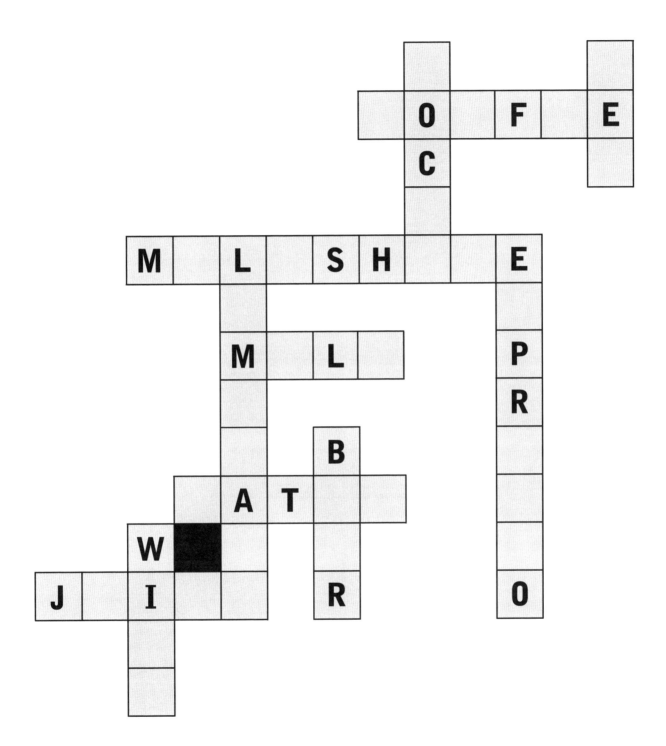

Fill in the names of trees.

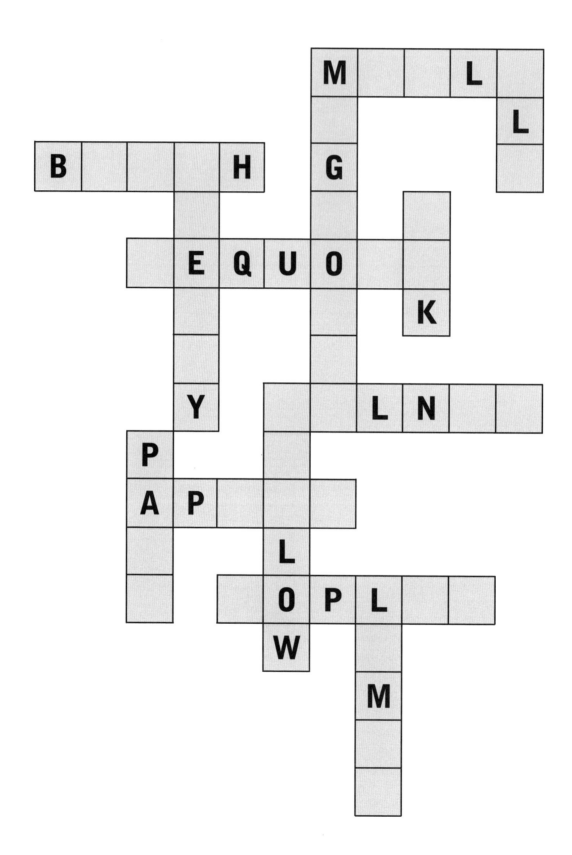

TARGET AREA 1: Word Formation

Crossword Fill-Ins

DIRECTIONS: In this crossword, some letters are already filled in. Complete the crossword with letters to form your own words. There are many possible answers. See **CLUES** for help.

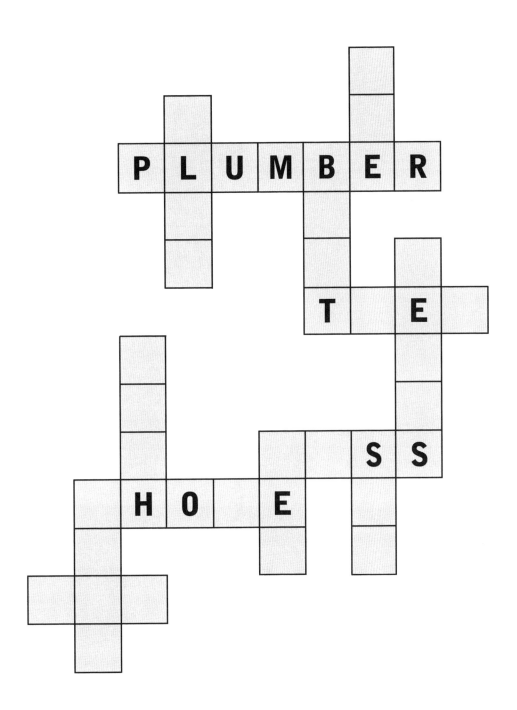

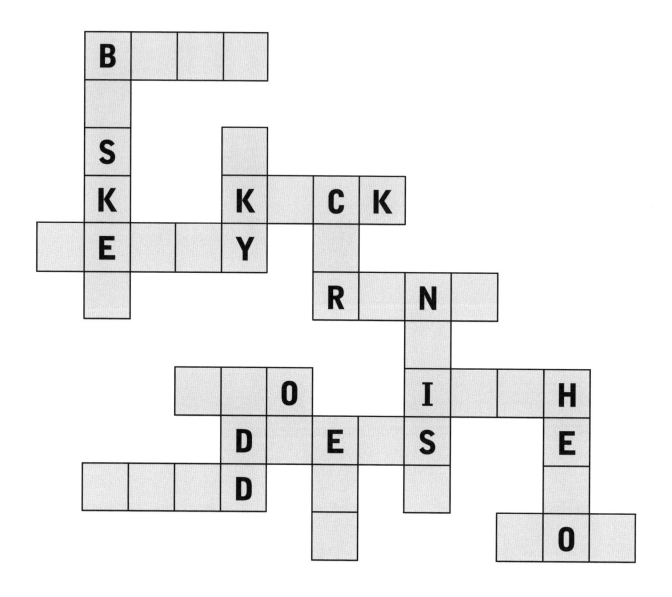

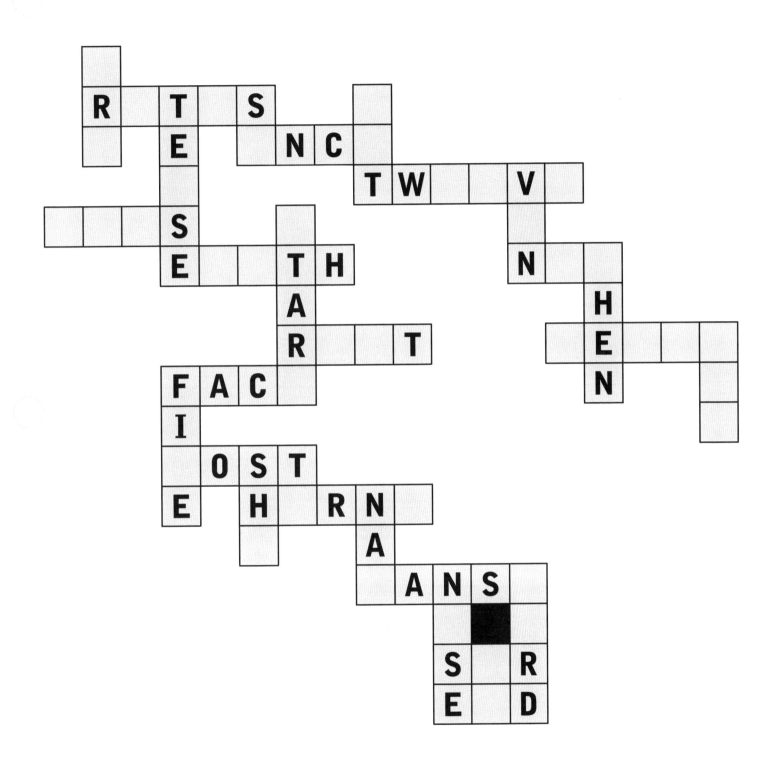

TARGET AREA 1: Word Formation

Mini-Grids

DIRECTIONS: Fill in the grids with your own words to make a puzzle that reads across and down. There are many possible answers. See **CLUES** *for help.*

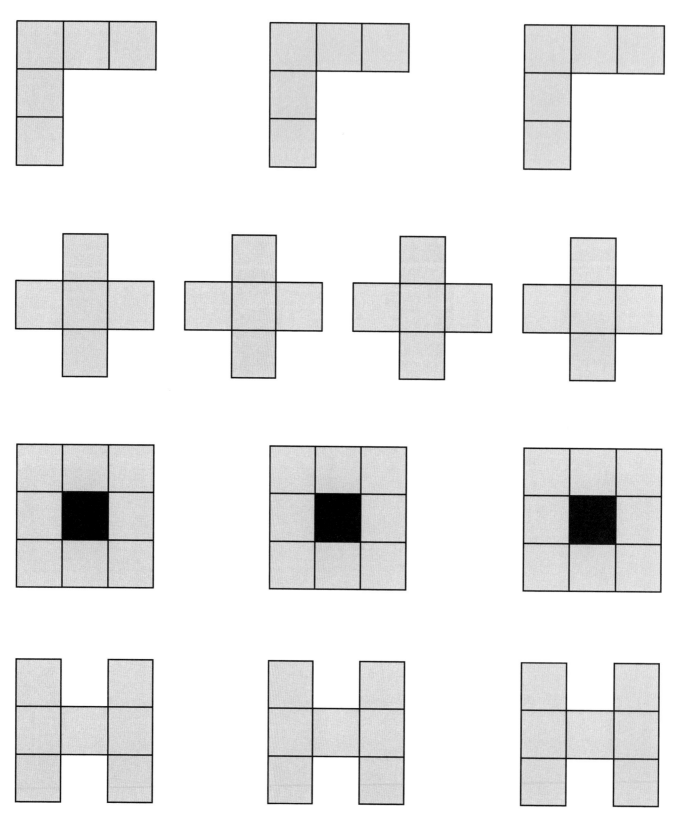

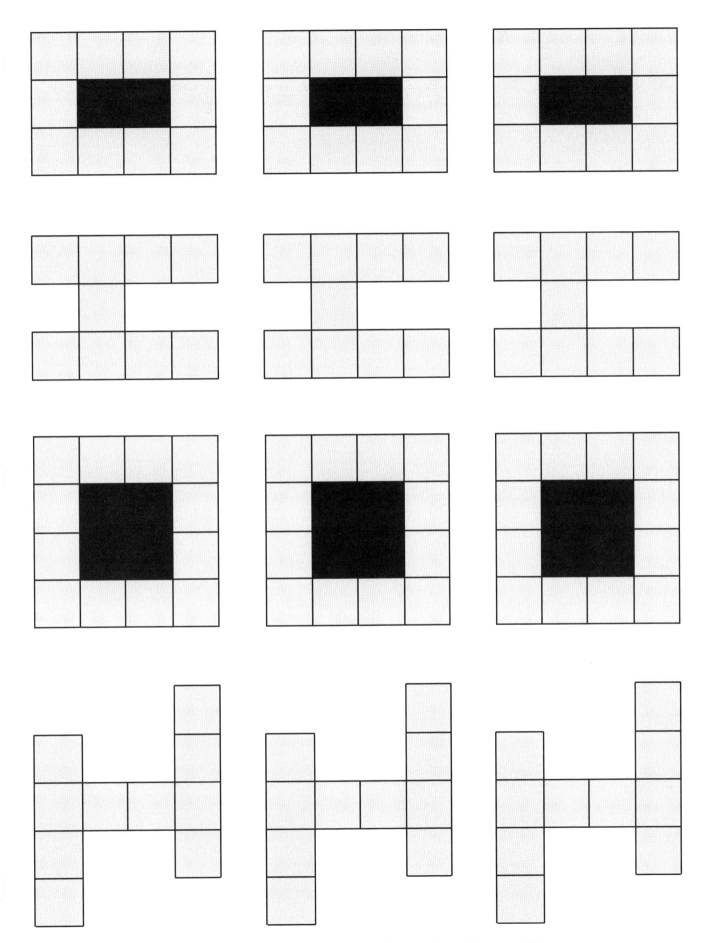

TARGET AREA 1: Word Formation

Crossword Grids

DIRECTIONS: Fill in the grids with all your own words to make a crossword reading across and down. There are many possible answers. See **CLUES** for help.

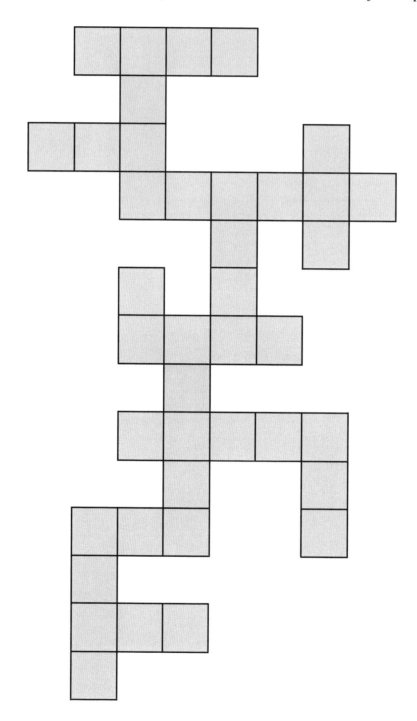

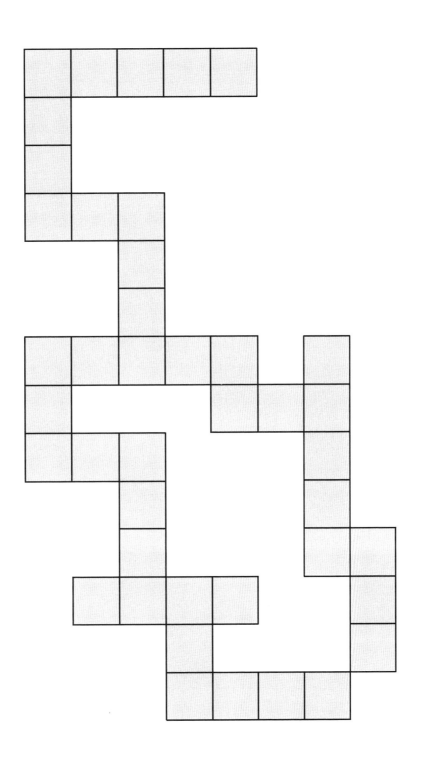

TARGET AREA 2:
Familiar Phrases

TARGET AREA 2: Familiar Phrases　　　　　Related Matches

DIRECTIONS: This page contains two items that go together. Complete the phrase on the left with a word from the column on the right. Write the number of the word that completes the phrase on the line. See **CLUES** for help.

eat and ____ 　　　　　　　1. shine

hugs and ____ 　　　　　　　2. vinegar

rise and ____ 　　　　　　　3. simple

vitamins and ____ 　　　　　4. kisses

odds and ____ 　　　　　　　5. tuck

oil and ____ 　　　　　　　　6. minerals

law and ____ 　　　　　　　　7. run

nip and ____ 　　　　　　　　8. order

stocks and ____ 　　　　　　9. ends

pure and ____ 　　　　　　　10. bonds

Add the fourth word in the four-word phrases.

here, there, and ____   1. pop

reading, writing, and ____   2. future

ear, nose, and ____   3. blue

snap, crackle, and ____   4. tomato

animal, vegetable, or ____   5. everywhere

red, white, and ____   6. delivered

bacon, lettuce, and ____   7. mineral

past, present, and ____   8. steal

signed, sealed, and ____   9. arithmetic

beg, borrow, or ____   10. throat

Match the words that can be opposites.

elevator   ____

out   ____

hair   ____

down   ____

dry ice   ____

shower   ____

buy   ____

land   ____

video   ____

king   ____

1. home run

2. across

3. sauna

4. rent

5. ace

6. take off

7. stairs

8. bald

9. bath

10. audio

Match the equipment with the profession.

gel ____   1. auctioneer

putter ____   2. insurance agent

Wall Street Journal ____   3. stylist

patent ____   4. cardiologist

gavel ____   5. landscaper

heart monitor ____   6. diver

mulch ____   7. inventor

policy ____   8. carpenter

snorkel ____   9. broker

C-clamp ____   10. golfer

Match the food with one of its ingredients.

hash browns ____

guacamole ____

pralines ____

coleslaw ____

soufflé ____

minestrone ____

bananas foster ____

macaroons ____

Greek salad ____

truffles ____

1. vegetables

2. chocolate

3. avocados

4. potatoes

5. ice cream

6. coconut

7. egg whites

8. nuts

9. cabbage

10. feta cheese

Match the famous couples.

Cinderella and ____   1. Eve

Beauty and the ____   2. Robin

Romeo and ____   3. Juliet

Adam and ____   4. Cleopatra

Hansel and ____   5. Prince Charming

Anthony and ____   6. Lois Lane

Dr. Jekyll and ____   7. Mr. Hyde

Batman and ____   8. Beast

Snow White and the ____   9. Gretel

Superman and ____   10. Seven Dwarfs

Match two words that rhyme with each other.

light ____

flute ____

go ____

bee ____

calf ____

trace ____

socks ____

June ____

meal ____

loop ____

1. feel

2. laugh

3. sea

4. boot

5. dough

6. soup

7. white

8. moon

9. base

10. box

Match the object with its category.

flannel _____   1. fabric

thistle _____   2. clothing

rottweiler _____   3. color

scallion _____   4. nut

pistachio _____   5. insect

polo _____   6. vegetable

mite _____   7. dog

kilt _____   8. plant

teal _____   9. animal

llama _____   10. sport

Match the object with its function.

jumper cables ____

kiln ____

floss ____

dam ____

sprinkles ____

iPod ____

herbs ____

canisters ____

intestines ____

air bags ____

1. decorate food

2. listen to music

3. aid in digestion

4. hold things

5. recharge a battery

6. flavor food

7. harden clay

8. clean between teeth

9. prevent injuries

10. control water flow

TARGET AREA 2: Familiar Phrases

Overlapping Phrases

DIRECTIONS: Each question consists of two phrases—one missing its last word and the other missing its first word. Write the one word that both phrases share on the line. See **CLUES** *for help.*

1. clean up your _____ service

2. be my _____ towels

3. we aim to _____ be seated

4. out of _____ in the court

5. jack in the _____ spring mattress

6. in the long _____ of the mill

7. put your foot _____ on your luck

8. the price is _____ up my alley

9. good _____ of the draw

10. take it _____ for you to say

11. the facts of _____ is too short

12. act your _____ before beauty

13. how do you _____ what I mean?

14. cut it _____ of the mouths of babes

15. do a double _____ my word for it

16. the sooner the _____ luck next time

17. don't give _____ to no good

18. make up your _____ if I join you

19. welcome to my _____ is where the heart is

20. been there, done _____ is no way to talk

21. call it a _____ care center

22. glad you could _____ and get it

23. need I say _____ than you'll ever know

24. get a good night's _____ tight

25. the life of the _____ of four

26. don't waste my _____ heals all wounds

27. a blank _____ it out

28. get up and _____ to your room

29. not by a long _____ in the arm

30. give a dirty _____ who's here

TARGET AREA 2: Familiar Phrases   Common Phrases

*DIRECTIONS: Each question is the first part of a common phrase. Complete the phrase with a word from the list at the bottom of the page. Each word should be used once. See **CLUES** for help.*

1. fame and _____

2. in sickness and in _____

3. raining cats and _____

4. fight tooth and _____

5. forgive and _____

6. aches and _____

7. through thick and _____

8. rules and _____

9. cut and _____

regulations	**paste**	**nail**
dogs	**fortune**	**pains**
forget	**thin**	**health**

1. too good to be _____

2. from rags to _____

3. X marks the _____

4. last but not _____

5. mind your own _____

6. on the tip of my _____

7. love at first _____

8. on the spur of the _____

9. a tough act to _____

10. lay down the _____

11. drive a hard _____

12. better safe than _____

business	moment	bargain
law	riches	least
true	sorry	spot
follow	tongue	sight

1. between a rock and a   _____

2. here today and   _____

3. in one ear and out   _____

4. square peg in a   _____

5. take it or   _____

6. sign on the   _____

7. first come,   _____

8. finders keepers,   _____

9. long time,   _____

10. save it for a   _____

leave it	**round hole**	**gone tomorrow**
the other	**hard place**	**losers weepers**
rainy day	**no see**	**first served**
dotted line		

TARGET AREA 2: Familiar Phrases   Alliterative Phrases

*DIRECTIONS: Each group shows part of a phrase that contains two words that begin with the same letter. The number of missing letters and a clue to its meaning are given. Fill in the missing letters. See **CLUES** for help.*

1. **r** ___ ___ ___   and   **r** ___ ___ ___
   type of music

2. **bl** ___ ___ ___   and   **bl** ___ ___
   colors of a bruise

3. **sp** ___ ___   and   **sp** ___ ___
   very clean

4. **tr** ___ ___ ___   or   **tr** ___ ___ ___
   Halloween greeting

5. **w** ___ ___ ___   and   **w** ___ ___ ___
   type of fabric that is easy to take care of

6. **st** ___ ___ ___   and   **st** ___ ___ ___ ___ ___
   pattern that makes up the American flag

7. **d** ___ ' ___   and   **d** ___ ___ ' ___ ___
   informal set of rules

8. **f** ___ ___ ___ ___   or   **f** ___ ___ ___ ___ ___
   either too much or too little of something

9. **n** ___ ___   or   **n** ___ ___ ___ ___

time to take action

---

10. **dr** ___ ___ ___   and   **dr** ___ ___ ___

if you do the first at a party, don't do the second

---

11. **s** ___ ___ ___ ___   and   **s** ___ ___ ___ ___

these are worn on your feet

---

12. **tr** ___ ___ ___   and   **tr** ___ ___

proven to be reliable

---

13. **b** ___ ___   and   **b** ___ ___ ___ ___ ___ ___ ___ ___

an alternative to a hotel

---

14. **r** ___ ___ ___ ___   of the   **r** ___ ___ ___

traffic laws

---

15. **r** ___ ___ ___   to   **r** ___ ___ ___ ___ ___

from poor to wealthy

---

16. **b** ___ ___ ___ ___   and   **b** ___ ___ ___ ___ ___

the basics of a sandwich

---

17. **s** ___ ___ ___   and   **s** ___ ___ ___ ___

out of danger

TARGET AREA 2: Familiar Phrases   Alliterative Terms

DIRECTIONS: Each group shows a phrase or compound word beginning with the same two letters. The number of missing letters and a clue to its meaning are given. Fill in the missing letters. See **CLUES** *for help.*

1. **b** ___ ___ ___   **b** ___ ___ ___ ___ ___ ___
   name for those born in the late 1940s, '50s, and '60s

_____

2. **b** ___ ___ ___   **b** ___ ___ ___ ___
   men can get this from drinking too much Budweiser

_____

3. **s** ___ ___ ___ ___ ___ ___ ___ ___ ___   **s** ___ ___ ___ ___
   fumes from other people's cigarettes

_____

4. **b** ___ ___ ___ ___ ___ **b** ___ ___
   type of insect that stings

_____

5. **m** ___ ___ ___ ___ **m** ___ ___ ___ ___
   one who tries to pair up other people

_____

6. **b** ___ ___ ___ ___   **b** ___ ___ ___ ___ ___
   the hole in everyone's tummy

_____

7. **c** ___ ___ ___ ___   **c** ___ ___
   means of transportation in San Francisco

8. s __ __ __ __ __   s __ __ __ __ __ __
they provide protection for U.S. presidents

9. c __ __ __ __ __ __ __ __   c __ __ __ __ __ __
local institution providing post–high school classes

10. c __ __ __ __ __ c __ __ __
popular refrigerated dessert often baked in a graham-cracker crust

11. f __ __ __ __ __   f __ __ __ __
food made from cooked strips of potato

12. h __ __ __ __   h __ __ __
time period before dinner when bars offer special prices

13. l __ __ __ __ __ __   l __ __ __
woman with the main role in a movie or play

14. b __ __ __ __   b __ __
recording device in the cockpit of planes

15. p __ __ __ __ __   p __ __ __
method of sending packages in the mail

16. p __ __   p __ __ __ __
habit someone has that really bothers you

17. **p** ___ ___ ___ ___   **p** ___ ___ ___ ___ ___ ___
someone who is very careful about spending money

---

18. **m** ___ ___ ___ ___ **m** ___ ___ ___ ___ ___ ___
key ingredient in s'mores

---

19. **s** ___ ___ ___ ___   **s** ___ ___ ___
piece of paper needed to return an item

---

20. **d** ___ ___ ___ ___ ___   **d** ___ ___ ___ ___ ___ ___
set-up in which a check goes right into your account

---

21. **s** ___ ___ ___ ___ - **s** ___ ___
tourists often do this while on vacation

---

22. **m** ___ ___ ___ ___   **m** ___ ___ ___ ___ ___
type of investment funds

---

23. **s** ___ ___ ___ ___ ___   **s** ___ ___ ___ ___ ___ ___ ___
Uncle Sam takes money for this every paycheck

---

24. **s** ___ ___ ___ ___ ___ ___ ___ ___   **s** ___ ___ ___ ___
metal resistant to rust and corrosion

---

25. **s** ___ ___ ___ ___ **s** ___ ___ ___
comfortable clothing to wear when exercising

26. **A** ___ ___ ___ ___ ___ ___   **A** ___ ___ ___ ___ ___
ceremony in which Oscars are given out

---

27. **t** ___ ___ ___ ___ ___   **t** ___ ___ ___ ___ ___ ___
words that are hard to say together fast

---

28. **t** ___ ___   **t** ___ ___ ___ ___
vehicle used to move vehicles that can't be driven

---

29. **v** ___ ___ ___   **v** ___ ___ ___ ___
just the same the other way around

---

30. **w** ___ ___ ___ ___   **w** ___ ___ ___ ___
healthy flour made from the entire grain

---

31. **h** ___ ___ ___   **h** ___ ___ ___
part of a clock face

---

32. **p** ___ ___ ___   **p** ___ ___ ___ ___ ___
pretend to be asleep

---

33. **b** ___ ___   **b** ___ ___ ___ ___ ___
ordinary name for halitosis

---

34. **s** ___ ___ ___ ___ ___   **s** ___ ___ ___ ___
so afraid you can't move

TARGET AREA 2: Familiar Phrases Words in Common

*DIRECTIONS: Each grouping has four phrases that have one word in common. Each phrase shows the missing letter and a clue to its meaning. Fill in the missing letters. See **CLUES** for help.*

1. | All phrases include the word **TIME.**

___ ___ ___ ___ **time**
more pay for more work

___ ___ ___ ___ ___ ___ ___ ___   ___ **time**
the first four words in many fairy tales

___ ___ ___ ___ ___ ___ ___ ___ **time**
don't hurry

___ ___ ___ **time** ___ ___ ___ ___ ___
what young children like to hear before sleeping

2. | All phrases contain the word **SHOW.**

___ ___ **- show**
someone who is expected but doesn't appear

___ ___ ___ ___ ___ ___ ___ **show**
event in which people model clothing

show ___ ___ ___ ___ ___ ___ ___
talk about an item you brought for others to see

___ ___ ___ ___ **show**
Jeopardy or Wheel of Fortune

3. All phrases contain the word **EYE.**

eye __ __ __ __ __ __ __

someone who sees something as it happens

__ __ __ __ ' __   **eye**

center of a target

__ __ __ __ __ __ __   **eye**

investigator hired by someone

__ __ __ **eye**   __ __   **eye**

agree with someone on an issue

__ __ __ __ __ - **eye** __   __ __ __ __

vegetable

---

4. All phrases contain the word **HOUSE.**

__ __   __ __ __   **house**

get something free, such as a drink or a sample

__ __ __ __ **house**

expensive top-floor living quarters

__ __ __ __ __ **house**

where trials take place

house __ __ __ __ __ __ __

a celebration after moving to a new place

__ __ __ __ **house**

place where inventory is stored

5. | All phrases contain the word **TURN.** |

turn __ __ __ __   __   __ __ __   __ __ __ __

make a positive change for yourself

__ __ __ __   __ __ __ **turn**

what you do when you are not getting a good night's sleep

__ __ __ __ **turn** __ __

an interesting and exciting book

turn __ __ __   __ __ __ __ __   __ __ __ __ __ __

do not retaliate when someone does something mean to you

__ __ __ __   __ __ __ __ **turn**

stand patiently in a line

6. | All phrases contain the word **TOP.** |

top __ __   __ __ __   __ __ __ __ __ __

Irish greeting

top __ __ __ __ __ __

something very confidential and important

top __ __ __ __

outer garment for cool days

__ __ __ **top**

name for a small portable computer

top __ __   __ __ __   __ __ __ __

the best quality there is

7. | All phrases contain the word **BREAK.**

__ __ __ __ __ __ **break**

time out during a working day

__ __ __ __ __ __ __ **break** __ __

a switch to stop the flow of electricity

break __ __ __ __

make as much money as you spend

break __ __ __ __

this is often said to stop people who are fighting

break __ __ __ __ __ __

make the first move to meet someone

___

8. | All phrases contain the word **LONG.**

__ __ __ __ __ **long** __ __ __ __

insects with long appendages

long __ __ __ __ __ __ __ __

worker who loads and unloads ships

long– __ __ __ __ __ __

describes someone who speaks lots and says little

Long __ __ __ __ __ __

Manhattan is near here

long __ __ __ __ __

underwear for a cold climate

TARGET AREA 2: Familiar Phrases   Rhyming Words

*DIRECTIONS: Each group has a phrase or compound word in which the two words rhyme. Each phrase shows the number of missing letters and a clue to its meaning. Fill in the missing letters. See **CLUES** for help.*

1. ___ ___ **ime** ___ **ime**
main TV show hours

9. ___ **ack** ___ ___ **ack**
retrace your footsteps

2. ___ **umpty** ___ **umpty**
he fell in a nursery rhyme

10. ___ **ed** ___ ___ ___ **ead**
covering over a blanket

3. ___ ___ **ack** ___ **ack**
card game

11. ___ **ook** ___ **ook**
it contains recipes

4. ___ ___ **ip -** ___ ___ **ops**
type of sandal

12. ___ ___ **and** ___ ___ **and**
seats overlooking a parade

5. ___ **ight-** ___ **ight**
it helps you see in the dark

13. ___ **ishy -** ___ **ashy**
can't make up one's mind

6. ___ **ir** ___ **are**
cost of traveling by plane

14. ___ ___ **ick** ___ ___ **ick**
movie appealing to women

7. ___ **ender** ___ **ender**
small car accident

15. ___ ___ **ite** ___ ___ **ight**
the one in shining armor

8. ___ **ooper -** ___ ___ **ooper**
used to clean up after a dog

16. ___ ___ **ue** ___ ___ **ue**
dedicated and devoted

Workbook for Cognitive Skills copyright © Susan Howell Brubaker 2009

TARGET AREA 2: Familiar Phrases

Clichés

DIRECTIONS: *Each phrase is missing its first word. Complete the phrase with a word from the list at the bottom of the page. Each word should be used once. See* **CLUES** *for help.*

1. _____ the beans

2. _____ the bullet

3. _____ the dots

4. _____ the walls

5. _____ the buck

6. _____ the fifth

7. _____ the drain

8. _____ the ice

9. _____ the scenes

10. _____ the field

11. _____ the whip

12. _____ the hatchet

13. _____ the jackpot

14. _____ the ball

15. _____ the plank

16. _____ the knot

17. _____ the difference

18. _____ the question

bury	**crack**	**climb**	**drop**
down	**behind**	**hit**	**bite**
walk	**spill**	**take**	**split**
break	**pop**	**pass**	**tie**
connect	**play**		

1. _____ in the door
2. _____ in the bud
3. _____ in the rough
4. _____ in the new year
5. _____ in the closet
6. _____ in the hole
7. _____ in the towel
8. _____ in the neck
9. _____ in a blue moon
10. _____ in a million

11. _____ of the party
12. _____ of the press
13. _____ of the road
14. _____ of the draw
15. _____ of the iceberg
16. _____ of the ways
17. _____ of the peace
18. _____ of the blue
19. _____ of the game
20. _____ of the fittest

out	throw	luck	diamond
nip	tip	skeleton	survival
ring	foot	life	ace
freedom	pain	name	middle
once	justice	one	parting

1. how now brown _____

2. in the _____ house

3. see you later _____

4. in a while _____

5. get your _____ s in order

6. _____ business

7. an _____ never forgets

8. _____ of approval

9. sly as a _____

10. pop goes the _____

11. a wild _____ chase

12. hit the _____ 's eye

13. a _____ in _____ 's clothing

14. when the _____ 's away, the _____ will play

15. March comes in like a _____ , out like a _____

16. strain at a _____ and swallow a _____

monkey	goose	bull	cat
wolf	lion	weasel	duck
fox	cow	elephant	mice
lamb	camel	crocodile	seal
alligator	dog	sheep	gnat

Workbook for Cognitive Skills copyright © Susan Howell Brubaker 2009

TARGET AREA 2: Familiar Phrases   Category Phrases

DIRECTIONS: Each grouping has four phrases that are each missing a word. The category in which the word belongs and its number of letters are also shown. Fill in the missing letters. See CLUES for help.

1. **FOODS**

   the best thing since sliced   __ __ __ __ __

   it's not my cup of   __ __ __

   the   __ __ __ __ __   of my eye

   a   __ __ __ __ __   to your success

2. **MEN'S NAMES**

   __ __ __ __   of Rights

   Peeping   __ __ __

   __ __ __ __ - o' - lantern

   __ __ __ bing for apples

3. **ANIMALS**

   let the   __ __ __   out of the bag

   __ __ __ __   in your throat

   take the   __ __ __ __   by the horns

   straight from the   __ __ __ __ __ 's   mouth

Workbook for Cognitive Skills copyright © Susan Howell Brubaker 2009

4. **CLOTHING**

a Freudian ___ ___ ___ ___

handle with kid ___ ___ ___ ___ ___ ___

hot under the ___ ___ ___ ___ ___ ___

fly by the seat of your ___ ___ ___ ___ ___

if the ___ ___ ___ ___ fits, wear it

---

5. **PARTS OF THE BODY**

put your best ___ ___ ___ ___ forward

keep a stiff upper ___ ___ ___

___ ___ ___ ___ over heels in love

get to the ___ ___ ___ ___ ___ of the matter

talk until you're blue in the ___ ___ ___ ___

---

6. **COLORS**

the jolly ___ ___ ___ ___ ___ giant

follow the ___ ___ ___ ___ ___ ___ brick road

little ___ ___ ___ ___ ___ lie

roll out the ___ ___ ___ carpet

pot of ___ ___ ___ ___ at the end of the rainbow

TARGET AREA 2: Familiar Phrases

Abbreviations to Words

DIRECTIONS: Write the abbreviations that are described on the numbered lines. Transfer the letter to its numbered line below it. If you answer correctly, the line will spell out a word or phrase. See **CLUES** for help.

___ ___   abbreviation of the smallest state in the United States
1   2

___ ___   person in the U.S. armed forces
3   4

___ ___   an organization working to keep peace in the world
5   6

___ ___   direction to go to get from Chicago to Miami
7   8

___ ___   general college degree completed after four years
9   10

___ ___ ___   ___ ___ ___ ___ ___ ___ ___ ___
9 2 3   9 5 7 4 6 8 7 7

___ ___ ___   America
 1   2   3

___ ___ ___   inscription on a tombstone
 4   5   6

___ ___ ___   how a package arrives if you need to pay for it
 7   8   9

___ ___ ___   government agency that looks into crime
 10   11   12

___ ___ ___   agreement that you will pay someone back
 13   14   15

___ ___ ___ ___ ___ ___ ___ ___ ___
 7   3   4   9   11   14   3   4   9

___ ___ ___ ___   term expressing pleasure at the end of the workweek
 1   2   3   4

___ ___ ___   network TV station
 5   6   7

___ ___ ___   Boston is in this time zone
 8   9   10

___ ___ ___   "smart" government organization
 11   12   13

___ ___ ___ ___ ___ ___ ___ ___ ___
 4   13   5   10   13   9   1   12   7

TARGET AREA 2: Familiar Phrases   Motivating Quotes

*DIRECTIONS: The motivating quotes are missing the first letters of most of their words. Fill in the missing letters so the quote makes sense. See **CLUES** for help.*

1. ___ aughter ___ s ___ he ___ est ___ edicine.

2. ___ on't ___ ive ___ p ___ nd ___ on't ___ ive ___ n.

3. ___ othing ___ entured, ___ othing ___ ained.

4. ___ ou ___ re a ___ onderful ___ riginal.

5. ___ on't ___ ind ___ ault. ___ ind a ___ emedy.

6. ___ ife ___ s ___ ull ___ f ___ hoices.

7. ___ mile ___ nd ___ he ___ orld ___ miles ___ ith ___ ou.

8. ___ here ___ re ___ o ___ umb ___ uestions.

9. ___ hen ___ ne ___ oor ___ loses, ___ nother ___ ne ___ pens.

10. ___ ount   ___ our   ___ lessings,   ___ ot   ___ our   ___ roubles.

11. ___ f   ___ ou   ___ est,   ___ ou   ___ ust.

12. ___ omorrow   ___ s   ___ nother   ___ ay.

13. ___ on't   ___ ook   ___ ack,   ___ ook   ___ orward.

14. ___ hallenge   ___ s   ___ pportunity   ___ n   ___ ork   ___ lothes.

15. ___ inners   ___ ever   ___ uit   ___ nd   ___ uitters   ___ ever   ___ in.

16. ___ augh   ___ nd   ___ he   ___ orld   ___ aughs   ___ ith   ___ ou.

17. ___ ook   ___ or   ___ pportunities,   ___ ot   ___ uarantees.

18. ___ here   ___ here's   a   ___ ill,   ___ here's   a   ___ ay.

19. ___ ttitude   ___ nd   ___ uccess   ___ o   ___ ogether.

20. A   ___ ay   ___ ithout   ___ aughter   ___ s   a   ___ ay   ___ asted.

TARGET AREA 2: Familiar Phrases   Incomplete Proverbs

*DIRECTIONS: Each proverb is missing most of its words. The first letter of each missing word is given. Write the rest of the word on the line. See **CLUES** for help.*

1. An   a _____   a   d _____   k _____

   the   d _____   a _____ .

_____

2. Don't   c _____   your   c _____

   b _____   they're   h _____ .

_____

3. No   n _____   is   g _____   n _____ .

_____

4. H _____   is   the   b _____   p _____ .

_____

5. A _____   s _____   bring

   M _____   f _____ .

_____

6. Don't   p _____   all   your   e _____

   in   one   b _____ .

_____

7. You   can't   j _____   a   b _____

   by   its   c _____ .

8. Two   h _____   are   b _____   than   one.

---

9. The   g _____   is   a _____   g _____
on   the   other   s _____   of   the   f _____ .

---

10. You   can't   t _____   an   o _____
d _____   new   t _____ .

---

11. A _____   speak   l _____   than   w _____ .

---

12. N _____   is   c _____   but
d _____   and   t _____ .

---

13. You   t _____   the   w _____
r _____   out   of   my   m _____ .

---

14. The   b _____   t _____   in   l _____
are   f _____ .

---

15. The   e _____   b _____   gets   the   w _____ .

16. A _____ makes the h _____

   grow f _____ .

---

17. P_____ in g _____ h _____

   shouldn't t _____ s _____ .

---

18. B _____ of a f _____

   f _____ t _____ .

---

19. A p _____ s _____ is a

   p _____ e _____ .

---

20. R_____ wasn't b _____ in a d _____ .

---

21. A r _____ s _____ g _____

   no m _____ .

---

22. All's f _____ in l _____ and w _____ .

---

23. Don't b _____ the h _____ that

   f _____ y _____ .

TARGET AREA 2: Familiar Phrases   Split Sayings

*DIRECTIONS: The words for the proverbs are at the bottom of each page. Each line represents one missing word and the line length gives a clue to the length of the missing word. The first word in a proverb is capitalized in the word list. Each word should be used once. Write the proverbs on the line. See **CLUES** for help.*

1. _____ _____ _____

   _____ _____ .

2. _____ _____

   _____ _____ .

3. _____ _____ _____ ,

   _____ _____ _____ .

dogs	leisure	no
haste	Let	place
home	lie	repent
in	like	sleeping
in	Marry	There's

4. _____   _____

_____ – _____

_____   _____   _____ .

5. _____   _____ ,

_____   _____ .

6. _____   _____ ,

_____   _____   _____ .

warm	law	of	tenths
his	madness	Possession	heart
in	method	Cold	There's
is	nine	the	hands

7. _____   _____   _____

_____   _____ .

8. _____   _____   _____

_____   _____ .

9. _____   _____   _____ .

said	stranger	than	pay	It's
is	than	done	fiction	
Crime	doesn't	Truth	easier	

TARGET AREA 2: Familiar Phrases

*DIRECTIONS: Write the words from the sayings at the bottom of the page into the crossword grids. Each phrase fits into one grid. See **CLUES** for help.*

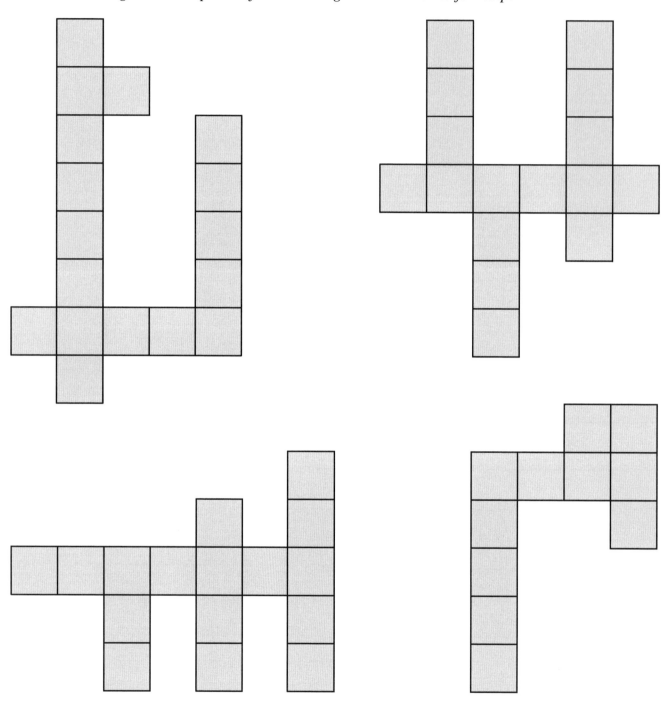

read between the lines

new lease on life

leave no stone unturned

better late than never

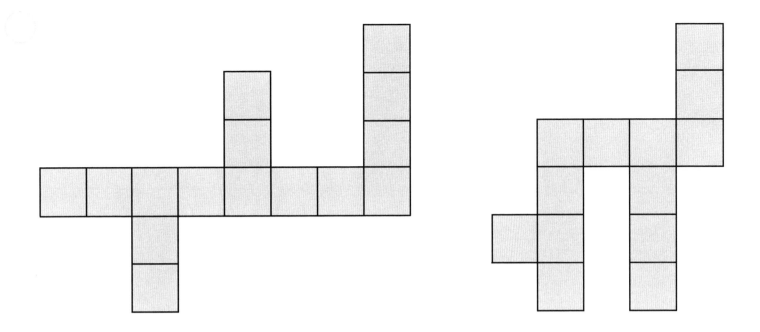

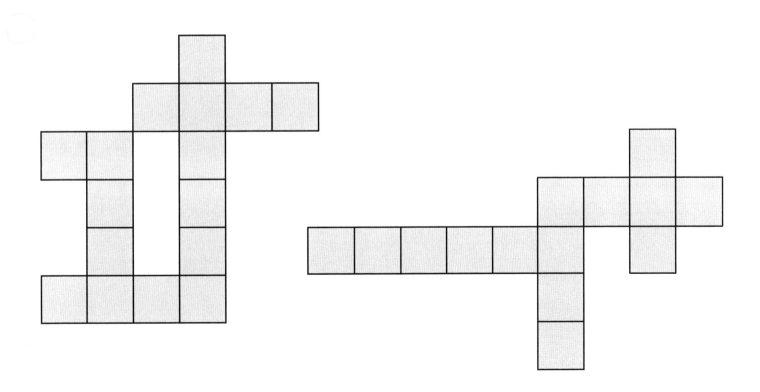

get your act together

beauty is only skin deep

look before you leap

life in the fast lane

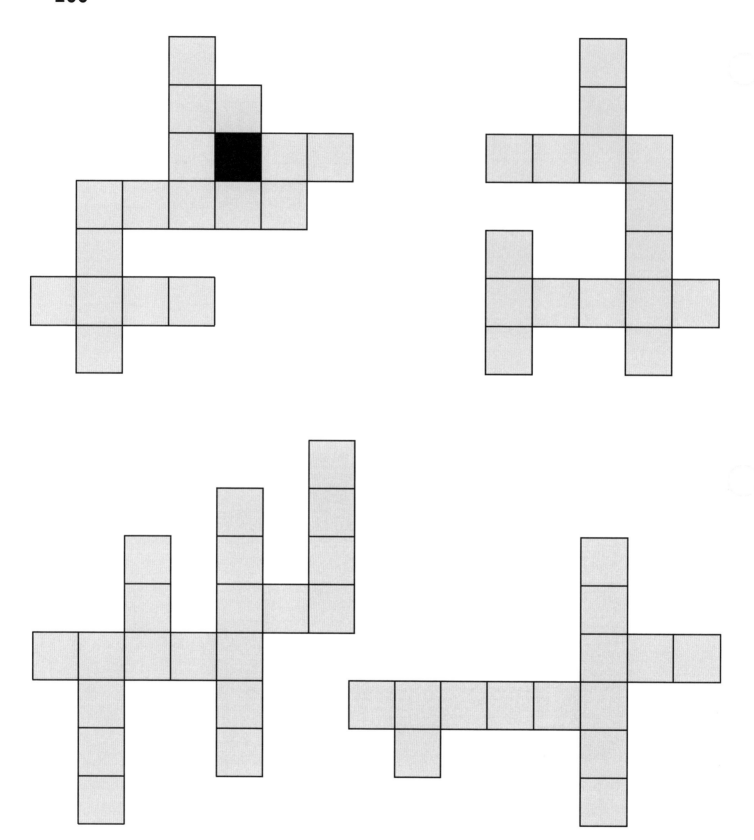

buckle up for safety

every rose has its thorn

your guess is as good as mine

take the bitter with the sweet

TARGET AREA 2: Familiar Phrases

Completion Word Search

DIRECTIONS: *The words you are to find in the grid below are described on the next page. The first letter and number of letters in the word are shown. Circle each word as you find it. See* **CLUES** *for help.*

```
F  T  S  D  C  M  E  H  O  B  O  V  X  A  L
R  H  A  F  D  A  O  P  O  S  S  I  B  L  E
A  O  L  C  C  E  G  U  X  O  K  M  B  L  G
G  U  V  F  C  S  P  E  N  T  A  C  L  E  W
I  S  A  W  R  H  D  O  T  T  E  D  E  G  L
L  A  T  J  S  T  A  N  D  A  A  D  K  I  M
E  N  I  O  A  C  F  I  S  W  Q  I  E  A  D
B  D  O  H  U  W  A  R  R  A  N  T  N  N  E
N  E  N  I  O  N  C  F  G  M  D  S  U  C  F
M  O  H  D  I  C  T  I  O  N  A  R  Y  E  E
F  A  T  A  H  C  S  A  K  J  M  N  L  Y  N
C  E  T  H  V  E  O  N  I  J  K  P  O  E  S
H  T  R  T  I  I  N  G  S  N  M  S  T  U  E
A  R  Y  C  E  N  O  D  D  I  T  Y  C  W  P
C  O  L  L  A  R  G  R  S  L  I  T  T  E  R
```

ACROSS

anything is   p __ __ __ __ __ __ __

look it up in the   d __ __ __ __ __ __ __ __ __

sign on the   d __ __ __ __ __   line

ring around the   c __ __ __ __ __

the pick of the   l __ __ __ __ __

I have a   w __ __ __ __ __ __   for your arrest

DOWN

I pledge   a __ __ __ __ __ __ __ __ __   to the flag

the   f __ __ __ __   speak for themselves

f __ __ __ __ __ __ ,   handle with care

the   d __ __ __ __ __ __   rests, your Honor

give to the   S __ __ __ __ __ __ __ __   Army

a picture is worth a   t __ __ __ __ __ __ __   words

DIAGONALLY   Left to right

be on your best   b __ __ __ __ __ __ __

the   c __ __ __ __ __ __ __   of the board

I had   n __ __ __ __ __ __   to do with it

as a   m __ __ __ __ __   of fact

I like the   s __ __ __ __ __   things in life

make a   m __ __ __ __ __ __ __   out of a molehill

TARGET AREA 2: Familiar Phrases   Celebrity Links

*DIRECTIONS: The three people in each group have something in common. Explain why they are grouped together. See **CLUES** for help.*

1. Brian Williams
    Charles Gibson   _____
    Katie Couric

2. Nemo
    Bambi   _____
    Dumbo

3. Noah
    Adam   _____
    Moses

4. Ralph Lauren
    Pierre Cardin   _____
    Calvin Klein

5. Beethoven
    Mozart   _____
    Handel

6. Naomi Campbell
    Tyra Banks   _____
    Heidi Klum

7. John Edwards
   John Kerry
   John McCain   _____

---

8. Renée Zellweger
   Halle Berry
   Julia Roberts   _____

---

9. Willie Wonka
   Hannibal Lecter
   Forrest Gump   _____

---

10. Smith & Wesson
    Black & Decker
    Barnes & Noble   _____

---

11. Jack Sprat
    Miss Muffet
    Georgie Porgie   _____

---

12. Julia Child
    Wolfgang Puck
    Emeril Lagasse   _____

---

13. Condoleezza Rice
    Nancy Pelosi
    Hillary Rodham Clinton   _____

14. Bon Jovi
    Rolling Stones   _____
    Beach Boys

15. Macbeth
    Hamlet   _____
    Othello

16. LeAnn Rimes
    Reba McEntire   _____
    Shania Twain

17. Evander Holyfield
    Muhammad Ali   _____
    Sugar Ray Leonard

18. Duncan Hines
    Sara Lee   _____
    Betty Crocker

19. Kirk & Michael Douglas
    Martin & Charlie Sheen   _____
    Donald & Kiefer Sutherland

20. Marion Jones
    Tonya Harding   _____
    Pete Rose

TARGET AREA 2: Familiar Phrases　　　　　　Celebrity Descriptions

*DIRECTIONS: Write the name of the famous person who is described. See **CLUES** for help.*

1. This man always wears a red shirt on the final day of a tournament. At the age of 30, he was the youngest golfer to have 50 PGA wins.

   _____

2. Known for her knowledge of everything domestic, this woman has her name on products for the home, a magazine, TV show, and books. Her time in prison for insider trading was national news.

   _____

3. "One small step for man, one giant step for mankind" was spoken on July 20, 1969, by this man as he walked on the moon.

   _____

4. This woman has the distinction of having the longest-running daytime TV talk show. Anything on her book club list is sure to sell millions of copies.

   _____

5. Born in 1706, this founding father of America has his picture on the hundred-dollar bill. He was also a scientist who invented the lightning rod, a stove, and bifocals that give him his distinctive look in portraits.

   _____

6. This actress is known for her beautiful voice. Her roles include Maria von Trapp in **The Sound of Music**, **Mary Poppins**, and more recently as the queen in **The Princess Diaries**.

_____

7. This creative man developed many cartoon characters. His theme parks still attract millions of visitors, and his animated films such as **Snow White** are classics.

_____

8. America celebrates the memory of this man on January 20. He was a Baptist minister whom we remember for his important work in civil rights.

_____

9. "You're fired" is the famous quote from his **Apprentice** TV reality show. He oversees a vast real estate empire centered in New York City.

_____

10. This actor got his start on TV's **Rawhide**. He played Dirty Harry, was mayor of Carmel, CA, and is an award-winning director and producer.

_____

11. This man is next-in-line after his father to become king of England. His mother was killed in a Paris car crash.

_____

12. This Dutch impressionist artist with one ear led an unhappy life. His original paintings now sell for millions of dollars.

_____

13. He is the first African American to run for president. He beat the first woman to run to get his party's nomination.

_____

14. This man is often referred to as the world's wealthiest person. He is the founder and owner of Microsoft Corporation.

_____

15. Bunnies are his trademark. He started the Playboy Club and has lived a life of wealth, women, and parties.

_____

16. She started with a cable TV show called **30 Minute Meals.** In 2006 she started hosting her own network talk show combining celebrities, information, and cooking.

_____

17. Two of this young-looking man's most popular TV jobs were hosting **American Bandstand** and New Year's Eve in New York City. He has worked hard to recover from a 2004 stroke.

_____

TARGET AREA 2: Familiar Phrases   First Names

*DIRECTIONS: The three people in each group have the same first name. Write that name on the line. See **CLUES** for help.*

1. _____
Doe
Eyre
Seymour

2. _____
Frost
Redford
De Niro

3. _____
Grisham
Travolta
McCain

4. _____
Stiller
Kingsley
Affleck

5. _____
Phil
Ruth
Scholl

6. _____
–Kate Olsen
Queen of Scots
Tyler Moore

7. _____

Burnett

King

Channing

8. _____

Lewis

Springer

Seinfeld

9. _____

Savage

Astaire

Flintstone

10. _____

Buffett

Carter

Smits

11. _____

Caine

Moore

Jordan

12. _____

Barker

Newhart

Dylan

13. _____

Foreman

Clooney

Bernard Shaw

14. _____

Dickens

Schwab

Darwin

15. _____

Harvey

Newman

Revere

16. _____

Crystal

Joel

Graham

17. _____

Lopez

Aniston

Garner

18. _____

Seagal

Spielberg

Colbert

19. _____

Sutherland

Rumsfeld

Duck

20. _____

Rodman

Quaid

Miller

TARGET AREA 2: Familiar Phrases

Last Names

*DIRECTIONS: The three people in each group have the same last name. Write that name on the line. See **CLUES** for help.*

1. Henry
   Harrison
   Gerald
   _____

2. Woody
   Ethan
   Tim
   _____

3. B.B.
   Larry
   Coretta Scott
   _____

4. Kathleen
   Tina
   Ted
   _____

5. Captain John
   Anna Nicole
   Will
   _____

6. Gary
   Alice
   Anderson
   _____

7. Jamie
   Vivica A.
   Michael J.

   _____

8. Mister
   Ginger
   Kenny

   _____

9. Jesse
   Samuel L.
   Reggie

   _____

10. Vanessa
    Robin
    Serena

    _____

11. Hugh
    Cary
    Ulysses S.

    _____

12. Helen Gurley
    Unsinkable Molly
    Buster

    _____

13. Rod
    Martha
    Jon

    _____

14. Laura
    Barbara
    George

    _____

15. Carly
    Neil
    Paul

    _____

16. Franklin
    Theodore
    Eleanor

    _____

17. Quincy
    Norah
    Catherine Zeta-

    _____

18. Vanna
    Betty
    Snow

    _____

19. Harpo
    Chico
    Groucho

    _____

20. Jessica
    Homer
    O.J.

    _____

TARGET AREA 2: Familiar Phrases   Incomplete Names

DIRECTIONS: Each grouping lists a category of people. Fill in either the first or last name of the person who fits the description. See **CLUES** *for help.*

1. | FEMALE SINGERS |

_____ Midler

_____ Streisand

Mariah _____

Celine _____

Aretha _____

3. | MALE SINGERS |

_____ Sinatra

_____ Manilow

_____ Springsteen

Stevie _____

Justin _____

2. | SPORTS FIGURES |

_____ Gretsky

_____ Gehrig

Lance _____

Shaquille _____

Magic _____

4. | PAST PRESIDENTS |

_____ Nixon

_____ Clinton

_____ Kennedy

Ronald _____

Abraham _____

5. ACTORS

_____ Depp

_____ Nicholson

Tom _____

Dustin _____

Denzel _____

8. ACTRESSES

_____ Hepburn

_____ Kidman

Angelina _____

Meryl _____

Halle _____

6. TV PERSONALITIES

_____ Seacrest

_____ Letterman

Regis _____

Ellen _____

Conan _____

9. WRITERS

_____ Crichton

_____ Twain

_____ Hemingway

J. K. _____

Danielle _____

7. MALE MOVIE CHARACTERS

_____ Potter

_____ Bond

Darth _____

Rhett _____

Indiana _____

10. PEOPLE IN HISTORY

_____ Churchill

_____ da Vinci

_____ Einstein

Mahatma _____

Ludwig van _____

TARGET AREA 2: Familiar Phrases   Literal Phrases

DIRECTIONS: Each group of letters represents a familiar phrase. Figure out the phrase by looking at the arrangement of the letters and words and interpreting them in a literal way. For example, if the word town *were written vertically or going down, the phrase would be* downtown. *See* **CLUES** *for help.*

1. MEsSAGes   _____

2. E   E
   A   A
   R   R
   T   T
   H   H   _____

3. busines   _____

4. 35 SAFETY 36   _____

5. COF   FEE   _____

6. EVERYrightTHING   _____

7. SLEEPING
   THE JOB   _____

8. MA ✓ IL   _____

9. DEATH   LIFE   _____

10. TAKE 1   BEDTIME   _____

11. pAI**NS**   _____

12. love ⟶ sight
            sight   _____

13. oHOnLEe   _____

      ↓
14. FOLD FOLD FOLD   _____

15.   WAIT
    HAND FOOT   _____

16. SALE SALE
    SALE SALE   _____

17. EVER
    EVER
    EVER
    EVER DAY

    _____

18. PO fish ND

    _____

19. I right I

    _____

20. ARREST
    YOU'RE

    _____

21. PARK PARK

    _____

22. C C
    GARAGE
    R R

    _____

23. THE BELT
         HIT

    _____

24. lang4uage

    _____

25. fapplauseof

    _____

TARGET AREA 3:
Definition Usage

TARGET AREA 3: Definition Usage   Defined Times Two

*DIRECTIONS: Each grouping has two definitions for the same word. Write the word that fits both on the line. See **CLUES** for help.*

1. title for a single woman

   fail to catch a ball; hit or . . .   _____

2. building in which to shop

   put things away until you need them   _____

3. the shore of a river

   institution that deals in money   _____

4. decide voluntarily to stop eating

   at a high rate of speed   _____

5. not ill; feeling fine

   source of natural ground water   _____

6. small mammal that flies at night

   what baseball players swing   _____

7. feel more than chilly

   mild illness

   _____

8. high part of an iceberg

   extra money given for good service

   _____

9. one of four suits in a card deck

   organization or association

   _____

10. main part of a tree

    name for an elephant's nose

    _____

11. a round object does this

    these may be served instead of bread

    _____

12. hard covering at the end of a finger

    thin metal piece with a flat top

    _____

13. music of the '50s and '60s

    large stone

    _____

14. players in a Broadway production

    protection for a broken bone

    _____

TARGET AREA 3: Definition Usage   Defined Times Three

*DIRECTIONS: Each grouping has three different definitions for the same word. Write the word that fits all three on the line. See **CLUES** for help.*

1. the sound from a phone

   a type of jewelry

   a circle

   The word is: _____

---

2. to make your voice louder

   to care for children until they are grown

   an increase in salary

   The word is: _____

---

3. to throw a ball to a batter

   a black, tarry substance

   to set up a tent

   The word is: _____

---

4. to organize in order

   a tool to smooth and shape nails

   to send in your 1040

   The word is: _____

5. a block of soap or chocolate

   a place where drinks are served

   a code on products

   The word is: _____

---

6. to look at

   to be careful

   a timepiece

   The word is: _____

---

7. to push down on something

   to use an iron

   a name for reporters

   The word is: _____

---

8. a place to swim

   to put in a common fund

   a table game

   The word is: _____

---

9. an expensive theater seat

   to fight with your fists

   a container

   The word is: _____

10. very thin and delicate

   money charged for a crime

   very good

   The word is: _____

---

11. to not fail

   a free ticket

   a football maneuver

   The word is: _____

---

12. to bend in a direction

   without much fat

   to use for support

   The word is: _____

---

13. to lubricate

   an ingredient in Italian dressing

   a type of paint

   The word is: _____

---

14. a car brand

   the substance in a thermometer

   a planet

   The word is: _____

15. a flat piece of wood

    a playing surface for some games

    to get on a plane

    The word is: _____

---

16. a social engagement

    a specific point on a calendar

    a small fruit

    The word is: _____

---

17. to hit again and again

    a place for homeless pets

    a unit of measure

    The word is: _____

---

18. to close tightly

    an official type of raised emblem

    water animal with flippers

    The word is: _____

TARGET AREA 3: Definition Usage   Alphabet Elimination

*DIRECTIONS: Fill in the letter blanks to complete each word. If you have completed the words correctly, all the letters of the alphabet will be used **one** time. See **CLUES** for help.*

| A B C D E F G H I J K L M N O P Q R S T U V W X Y Z |

1. y ___ s ___ er ___ a ___   the day before today

2. ___ nter ___ ediate   between beginning and advanced

3. c ___ eeseb ___ r ___ er   specialty at McDonald's and Wendy's

4. e ___ ___ el ___ ent   the best rating or grade

5. ___ olu ___ tee ___   someone who gives free help

6. ___ quee ___ e   how to get toothpaste from a tube

7. ___ ___ odpec ___ er   a noisy bird

8. ___ an ___ uet   large meal for many people

9. ___ e ___ lous   be envious of someone or something

10. ___ er ___ orm   act in front of a group

A B C D E F G H I J K L M N O P Q R S T U V W X Y Z

1. ___ in ___ er ___ arten   class before first grade

2. a ___ et ___ ___ st   purple gem, February birthstone

3. ___ a ___ es   up and down movement of water

4. e ___ ___ a ___ or   imaginary line at the earth's center

5. ___ e ___ t   the one after this one

6. ste ___ i ___ i ___ e   make germ-free by boiling

7. ___ ui ___ e   liquid squeezed from a fruit

8. ___ ___ ___ ore   prior to now

9. ch ___ m ___ i ___ n   winner of a competition

10. h ___ lariou ___   very, very funny

A B C D E F G H I J K L M N O P Q R S T U V W X Y Z

1. ___ a ___ il ___   Mom, Dad, and all the kids

2. ___ a ___ ___ idat ___   person who runs for office

3. e ___ ___ ens ___ ve   costing a lot

4. ___ ig ___ tnin ___   it accompanies thunder

5. ___ ay ___ al ___   cross a street in the middle of traffic

6. b ___ a ___ il   South American country

7. ___ ue ___ ___ ion   an inquiry about something

8. ___ ea ___ er   animal that builds dams

9. s ___ bp ___ en ___   paper that requires you to appear in court

132

TARGET AREA 3: Definition Usage   Overlapped Words

*DIRECTIONS: A letter goes in each of the numbered squares. The numbers by the definition show which squares to put the letters in. The words will overlap by two letters. See **CLUES** for help.*

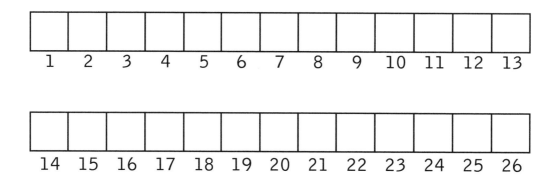

1	2	3	4	5	6	7	8	9	10	11	12	13

14	15	16	17	18	19	20	21	22	23	24	25	26

1 – 4   opposite of **slow**

3 – 7   keep looking at something

6 – 11   information to prepare a food dish

10 – 15   French word meaning **small** in size

14 – 20   insect that eats wood

19 – 22   examination

21 – 25   name for a small rock

24 – 26   opposite of **old**

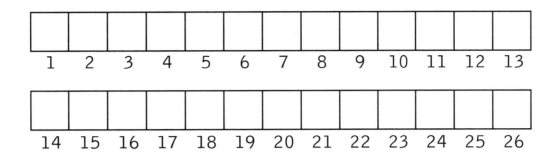

1	2	3	4	5	6	7	8	9	10	11	12	13

14	15	16	17	18	19	20	21	22	23	24	25	26

1 – 5	one-sixteenth of a pound
4 – 9	crunchy salad vegetable
8 – 10	type of bread with caraway seeds
9 – 12	365 days
11 – 16	take into custody by the police
15 – 20	place where horses live
19 – 23	it attaches to a dog's collar
22 – 26	not tall

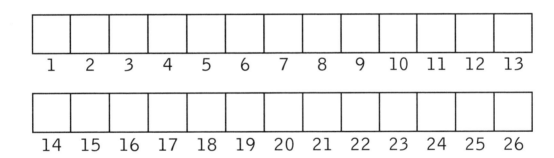

1	2	3	4	5	6	7	8	9	10	11	12	13

14	15	16	17	18	19	20	21	22	23	24	25	26

1 – 4	small green citrus fruit
3 – 6	you order food from this
5 – 9	a medical professional
8 – 13	look for something
12 – 17	place of worship
16 – 21	cheddar, swiss, or jack
20 – 25	opposite of **mild**
24 – 26	color of a **STOP** sign

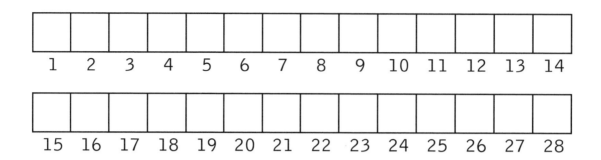

1	2	3	4	5	6	7	8	9	10	11	12	13	14

15	16	17	18	19	20	21	22	23	24	25	26	27	28

1 – 6   opposite of **male**

5 – 9   the lowest amount

8 – 11   opposite of **go**

10 – 13   pearly white gemstone

12 – 15   woman's singing voice

14 – 18   molar or bicuspid

17 – 20   opposite of **thick**

19 – 23   an alphabetized list

22 – 28   blow up; like a bomb

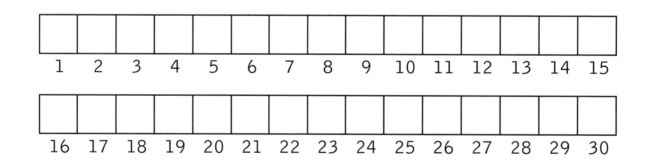

1	2	3	4	5	6	7	8	9	10	11	12	13	14	15

16	17	18	19	20	21	22	23	24	25	26	27	28	29	30

1 – 6   country north of the continental United States

5 – 9   move your body to music

8 – 13   an area below ground level

12 – 16   a pleasant smell

15 – 19   another one just like this one

18 – 26   ingredient in a Hershey bar

25 – 30   two- or four-person sport with a net

1	2	3	4	5	6	7	8	9	10	11	12	13	14	15

16	17	18	19	20	21	22	23	24	25	26	27	28	29	30

1 – 4	**Scrabble** or checkers
3 – 10	aspirin or pills
9 – 16	pendant or string of pearls
15 – 19	large stringed musical instrument
18 – 21	bread shape
20 – 25	scared or frightened
24 – 27	a thought that comes into your mind
26 – 30	the planet we live on

1	2	3	4	5	6	7	8	9	10	11	12	13	14	15	16

17	18	19	20	21	22	23	24	25	26	27	28	29	30	31	32

1 – 3	not cooked
2 – 6	not asleep
5 – 10	boarding place for animals
9 – 14	number after 10
13 – 20	container for a letter
19 – 23	fruit with a fuzzy skin
22 – 27	make a credit card purchase
26 – 32	country in central Europe

TARGET AREA 3: Definition Usage

Missing Ends

DIRECTIONS: *Add the correct letter to each end of the word shown to form the new word that is described. See CLUES for help.*

1. ___ hive ___   shake because of the cold

2. ___ raw ___   creep around on all fours

3. ___ do ___   an unpleasant smell

4. ___ ear ___   organ that pumps blood in the body

5. ___ hot ___   picture taken with a camera

6. ___ tea ___   evaporated water

7. ___ lie ___   person from another country or planet

8. ___ at ___   fence opening to walk through

9. ___ rows ___   sleepy or tired

10. ___ am ___   young sheep

11. ___ car ___   material to wrap around your neck

12. ___ r i b ___   something given to influence another

13. ___ e w e ___   valuable gem or mineral

14. ___ a s ___   it is worn at costume parties

15. ___ a c t o r ___   place where things are manufactured

16. ___ o d e ___   cattle show with contests

17. ___ s h e ___   what is left after a fire

18. ___ h u m ___   there is one on each hand

19. ___ h a s ___   run after someone

20. ___ n a m e ___   shiny paint or glaze

21. ___ a g e ___   money earned from a job

22. ___ a n d ___   black-and-white bear from China

23. ___ t o o ___   seat with three legs

24. ___ r o w ___   an upside-down smile

25. ___ w e e ___   opposite of **sour**

26. ___ i n ___   spouse of a queen

27. ___ e a r s ___   it heads a funeral procession

28. ___ t e e ___   a strong man-made metal

29. ___ h a n g ___   what is returned when you overpay

30. ___ b e ___   do as you are told

31. ___ c o w ___   unpleasant facial expression

32. ___ e d g e ___   pie-shaped pieces

33. ___ l a n e ___   Venus or Saturn

34. ___ o u t ___   your lips surround it

35. ___ h a m ___   short name for a winner

TARGET AREA 3: Definition Usage   **Missing Middles**

DIRECTIONS: Fill in the middle letters to complete each word. The number of missing letters and a description of the words is shown. See **CLUES** *for help.*

1. **a** ___ ___ ___ **a**
   Hawaiian greeting

_____

2. **b** ___ **b**
   babies wear this to catch food and drool

_____

3. **c** ___ ___ ___ ___ **c**
   person who reviews plays, shows, movies, etc.

_____

4. **d** ___ ___ ___ ___ ___ **d**
   the usual engagement rock

_____

5. **e** ___ ___ ___ **e**
   America's national bird

_____

6. **f** ___ ___ ___ ___ ___ ___ ___ **f**
   term for something that cannot be burned

_____

7. **g** ___ ___ ___ ___ ___ ___ ___ **g**
   animal that looks for his shadow in February

8. **h** ___ ___ **h**

opposite of **low**

---

9. **k** ___ ___ **k**

hit something with your foot

---

10. **l** ___ ___ ___ **l**

tag that gives information about a product

---

11. **m** ___ ___ ___ ___ **m**

cooking request between rare and well done

---

12. **n** ___ ___ ___ ___ ___ **n**

another word for an infant

---

13. **O** ___ ___ **o**

midwestern state

---

14. **p** ___ ___ ___ **p**

chubby; overweight

---

15. **r** ___ ___ ___ ___ **r**

fix something so it can be used

16. **s** ___ ___ ___ ___ ___ ___ **s**
    tool used to cut paper

    _____

17. **t** ___ ___ ___ ___ **t**
    where gargling takes place

    _____

18. **w** ___ ___ ___ ___ **w**
    glass opening used for ventilation and view

    _____

19. **X** ___ ___ ___ **x**
    company that produces copiers

    _____

20. **y** ___ ___ ___ ___ **y**
    every 365 days

    _____

21. **A** ___ ___ ___ ___ ___ **a**
    land of the free and home of the brave

    _____

22. **d** ___ ___ ___ ___ ___ **d**
    suffocated underwater

    _____

23. **n** ___ ___ ___ ___ ___ ___ ___ **n**
    bedtime clothing

24. **r** __ __ __ __ __ __**r**

type of handgun

_____

25. **s** __ __ __ __ __**s**

opposite of **failure**

_____

26. **w** __ __ __**w**

woman whose husband has died

_____

27. **t** __ __ __ __**t**

item a driver does not want to receive

_____

28. **e** __ __ __ __ __ __**e**

someone who works for you

_____

29. **m** __ __ __ __**m**

place where exhibits are formally displayed

_____

30. **r** __ __ __ __ __ __**r**

comfortable chair with a support for your feet

TARGET AREA 3: Definition Usage

DIRECTIONS: Fill in the missing letters to complete each word. The number of missing letters and a description of the word are shown. See **CLUES** *for help.*

1. **A** ___ ___ ___ ___ **a** ___ ___ **a**
   island country known for kangaroos

2. **B** ___ **bb** ___
   nickname for **Robert**

3. ___ **c c** ___ ___ ___ ___ ___ **c**
   odd or different from the norm

4. **d** ___ ___ ___ **d** ___ **d**
   separated into parts

5. **e** ___ **e** ___ ___ **e** ___ ___ ___
   situation that should be handled immediately

6. **f** ___ **f** ___ ___ **- f** ___ ___ ___
   number less than 100

7. **g** ___ **g g** ___ ___
   type of laughter

8. **h** ___ ___ **h** ___ ___ ___ **h** ___

mark text with a light bright color

___

9. **i** ___ **i** ___ ___ ___ **i** ___ ___

not real; a substitute for something

___

10. **l** ___ **ll** ___ ___ ___ ___

candy on a stick

___

11. **m** ___ ___ ___ **m** ___ **m**

the very most of something

___

12. **n** ___ **n** ___ ___ **n** ___ ___

something that doesn't have any meaning

___

13. ___ **o** ___ **o** ___ **o** ___ ___

the classic real estate board game

___

14. **p** ___ **pp** ___

young dog

___

15. ___ **r** ___ ___ ___ ___ **rr** ___

fruit for a Thanksgiving meal

16. ___ ___ ___ **s** ___ ___ **ss**
    enter someone's property illegally

17. **t** ___ ___ **t** ___ ___ ___ ___ **t** ___
    cleaner for your molars

18. **u** ___ **u** ___ **u** ___ ___
    out of the ordinary

19. ___ ___ **ww** ___ **w**
    a meeting, especially of Indian tribes

20. **e** ___ ___ **e** ___ ___ ___ ___ **e**
    very high in price

21. **i** ___ ___ **i** ___ ___ ___ **i** ___ ___
    formal request to attend an event

22. ___ ___ **rr** ___ ___ ___ ___ **r**
    give up, especially in war

23. ___ **ee** ___ ___ **e**
    sharp sewing tool

24. **d ___ dd ___**
nickname for a parent

_____

25. **___ ss ___ s ___**
help someone in a task

_____

26. **___ a ___ a ___ a**
yellow fruit you peel

_____

27. **___ i ___ i ___ i**
small two-piece bathing suit

_____

28. **n ___ n ___ ___ ___ ___ n**
a number

_____

29. **e ___ e ___ ___ ___ ___ e**
a way to get physically fit

_____

30. **t ___ tt ___ ___**
permanent body marking

TARGET AREA 3: Definition Usage

DIRECTIONS: *Rearrange the letter and word to make a new word. A definition of the new word is given. See* **CLUES** *for help.*

1. DRAPE + A = _____
   procession of bands and floats

2. BOARS + B = _____
   soak up liquid like a sponge

3. HEAR + C = _____
   stretch out your arm

4. PLEAD + D = _____
   use oars in a canoe

5. BOWL + E = _____
   joint in your arm

6. CRANE + F = _____
   European country

7. SAW + H = _____
   clean with soap and water

8. MORN + I = _____
   someone who is not of legal age

9. STEAL + B = _____
   home for horses

10. CAST + K = _____
    pile things on top of the other

11. TITLE + L = _____
    small or tiny

12. SINCE + T = _____
    mosquito or wasp

13. GEAR + N = _____
    name for a chain of mountains

14. STAB + O = _____
    brag about yourself

15. SUITE + S = _____
    what you use to blow your nose

16. ROOM + T = _____
    it makes boats run

17. SOME + U = _____
    small rodent that likes cheese

TARGET AREA 3: Definition Usage

Scrambled Triplets

*DIRECTIONS: Combine two letter blocks from the gray box to form words that fit each description. Write the word on the line. See **CLUES** for help.*

age	dol	ked	lar	ove
rch	rem	sco	voy	wic

1. _____ four quarters

   _____ trip or journey

   _____ take away

   _____ evil or bad

   _____ burn slightly

---

age	era	fin	gar	iod	ire	lve
mar	muf	oon	per	ret	ser	twe

2. _____ the correcting end of a pencil

   _____ place to keep a car

   _____ dark red color

   _____ breakfast pastry

   _____ number between 1 and 20

   _____ a mark to end a sentence

   _____ officially stop working

cer	cil	cue	der	dra	eal	ink
mur	nge	ora	pen	pes	res	shr

3. _____   citrus fruit

_____   writing utensil

_____   fabric covering for windows

_____   kill someone on purpose

_____   make something smaller in size

_____   save from danger

_____   popular breakfast food

buc	ale	eam	gen	hor	ice	kle
get	net	oxy	pol	exh	scr	for

4. _____   yell loudly

_____   we need this to breathe

_____   metal fastening on a belt

_____   stinging insect

_____   law enforcement agent

_____   breathe out

_____   fail to remember

TARGET AREA 3: Definition Usage   Double Meanings

DIRECTIONS: The four answers in each group fit the category in bold print. Each word can also be described by the description. Write the word that fits on the line. See CLUES for help.

1. **COLORS**

_____   _____
feel a little depressed   not very experienced

_____   _____
result of time in the sun   thorny flower

2. **FOODS**

_____   _____
go out together   an undesirable car

_____   _____
cut off dead branches   Halloween color

3. **CLOTHING**

_____   _____
hit with your bare hand   what a dog does when it is hot

_____   _____
lose your balance   make a knot

4. **THINGS IN KITCHEN CABINETS**

_____   _____
they correct vision   important baseball position

_____   _____
makes faces for a camera   roll a ball down an alley

Workbook for Cognitive Skills copyright © Susan Howell Brubaker 2009

TARGET AREA 3: Definition Usage   Fractured Words

DIRECTIONS: Each item gives the middle part of two words that belong together in the category. Add letters on the lines to complete the words. See CLUES for help.

1. **FOODS**

_____ e n c _____	_____ o a s _____	hot breakfast treat
_____ e a n _____	_____ u t t _____	sandwich filling
_____ r a w b _____	_____ c a _____	fruity dessert
_____ c k l _____	_____ e l i _____	hot dog topping
_____ a k _____	_____ e a n _____	BBQ side dish
_____ p p _____	_____ i d e _____	fruit drink
_____ h o c _____	_____ u d d _____	creamy dessert
_____ e d d _____	_____ e a _____	cereal
_____ a l _____	_____ e s s _____	ranch or Italian
_____ m p k _____	_____ i _____	seasonal dessert

2. | **CITIES AND THEIR STATES**

_____ osto _____   _____ achu _____   northeast

_____ opek _____   _____ ansa _____   west central

_____ enve _____   _____ olor _____   west

_____ eatt _____   _____ shin _____   northwest

_____ delp _____   _____ sylv _____   east

_____ rtla _____   _____ rego _____   northwest

_____ land _____   _____ lori _____   southeast

_____ hica _____   _____ llin _____   central

_____ hvil _____   _____ nnes _____   southeast

_____ olul _____   _____ awai _____   west

_____ lwau _____   _____ cons _____   north central

_____ alti _____   _____ ryla _____   east

_____ apol _____   _____ dian _____   central

_____ troi _____   _____ ichi _____   north central

TARGET AREA 3: Definition Usage   Letter Removal

DIRECTIONS: Work across the line in this exercise. On the first line, write a word that fits the definition below it. Remove one letter from that word to make a word that fits the definition on the next line. Write the letter that you subtracted from the first word on the third line. If you are correct, a food will be spelled reading down the third column. See **CLUES** *for help.*

1. _____   _____   ___ ___

   suffocate something   opposite of **father**

   _____   _____   ___ ___

   smell very badly   what you wash in

   _____   _____   ___ ___

   type of fir tree   piece of jewelry

   _____   _____   ___ ___

   heavy winter jacket   drive a car into a spot

   _____   _____   ___ ___

   man in armor   after dark

---

2. _____   _____   ___ ___

   your living place   garden tool

   _____   _____   ___ ___

   gave money for work   thin cushion

   _____   _____   ___ ___

   give temporarily   finish or stop

   _____   _____   ___ ___

   use your brain   slender

Workbook for Cognitive Skills copyright © Susan Howell Brubaker 2009

3. _____   _____   _____

      mark from a wound   automobile

   _____   _____   _____

      tidy and organized   tennis court part

   _____   _____   _____

      air transportation   window part

   _____   _____   _____

      hot water vapor   stalk of a flower

   _____   _____   _____

      prescription medicines   floor coverings

---

4. _____   _____   _____

      floor sweeper   section in a house

   _____   _____   _____

      stop a car   cook in an oven

   _____   _____   _____

      indebted to someone   married

   _____   _____   _____

      desire   small bug

   _____   _____   _____

      grassy areas   legal rules

   _____   _____   _____

      dangling fish food   baseball equipment

   _____   _____   _____

      underneath   force air out of your mouth

TARGET AREA 3: Definition Usage   Letter Transfers

DIRECTIONS: Write a word on the lines to fit the definition. Transfer the numbered letter to its correct spot on the line of consecutive numbers. If you are correct, the numbered line below will spell out a word. See CLUES for help.

1.

____ ____ ____
 4   5   2   use money to buy something

____ ____ ____ ____
 3   5   4   1   printed guides to an area

____ ____ ____ ____ ____
 1   6   5   3   4   postage square

____ ____ ____ ____
 8   5   3   1   sweet potatoes

____ ____ ____
 7   5   2   food for horses

____ ____ ____ ____ ____ ____ ____ ____
 1   2   3   4   5   6   7   8

2.

____ ____ ____ ____
 6   7   1   2   wrapped up in string or cord

____ ____ ____ ____
 6   1   1   9   someone between 13 and 19

____ ____ ____ ____
 4   8   5   6   cool-weather clothing

____ ____ ____ ____ ____
 3   9   7   6   1   bring together for a cause

____ ____ ____
 1   9   2   opposite of **begin**

____ ____ ____ ____ ____ ____ ____ ____ ____
 1   2   3   4   5   6   7   8   9

157

3.

$\underline{}\ \underline{}\ \underline{}\ \underline{}\ \underline{}$
8   11   3   9   12   lucky number

$\underline{}\ \underline{}\ \underline{}\ \underline{}\ \underline{}$
5   7   12   8   4   get the soap out

$\underline{}\ \underline{}\ \underline{}\ \underline{}$
2   7   4   13   try to lose weight

$\underline{}\ \underline{}\ \underline{}\ \underline{}\ \underline{}$
8   1   6   7   12   smooth and shiny fabric

$\underline{}\ \underline{}\ \underline{}\ \underline{}\ \underline{}\ \underline{}$
2   9   10   1   12   2   ask for strongly

$\underline{}\ \underline{}\ \underline{}\ \underline{}\ \underline{}\ \underline{}\ \underline{}\ \underline{}\ \underline{}\ \underline{}\ \underline{}\ \underline{}\ \underline{}$
1   2   3   4   5   6   7   8   9   10   11   12   13

4.

$\underline{}\ \underline{}\ \underline{}\ \underline{}\ \underline{}$
1   9   7   2   5   place to display photographs

$\underline{}\ \underline{}\ \underline{}\ \underline{}\ \underline{}$
9   10   1   11   3   the very minimum

$\underline{}\ \underline{}\ \underline{}\ \underline{}\ \underline{}\ \underline{}$
3   6   5   1   3   4   salad ingredient

$\underline{}\ \underline{}\ \underline{}\ \underline{}\ \underline{}$
11   5   8   9   10   facial expression

$\underline{}\ \underline{}\ \underline{}\ \underline{}\ \underline{}$
7   2   8   9   3   constructed

$\underline{}\ \underline{}\ \underline{}\ \underline{}\ \underline{}\ \underline{}\ \underline{}\ \underline{}\ \underline{}\ \underline{}\ \underline{}$
1   2   3   4   5   6   7   8   9   10   11

Continue as on previous pages. The transferred letters on the next four pages will spell out a word and its humorous definition.

1. ax with a short handle

$\underline{}_{7}\ \underline{}_{25}\ \underline{}_{14}\ \underline{}_{1}\ \underline{}_{15}\ \underline{}_{11}\ \underline{}_{22}$

Beauty and the . . .

$\underline{}_{17}\ \underline{}_{4}\ \underline{}_{16}\ \underline{}_{10}\ \underline{}_{26}$

breakfast, lunch, and dinner

$\underline{}_{3}\ \underline{}_{24}\ \underline{}_{6}\ \underline{}_{5}\ \underline{}_{23}$

brand name of a soft drink

$\underline{}_{19}\ \underline{}_{8}\ \underline{}_{20}\ \underline{}_{21}$

a fight between nations

$\underline{}_{12}\ \underline{}_{2}\ \underline{}_{9}$

matching jacket and pants

$\underline{}_{10}\ \underline{}_{18}\ \underline{}_{13}\ \underline{}_{26}$

run after someone

$\underline{}_{19}\ \underline{}_{7}\ \underline{}_{2}\ \underline{}_{23}\ \underline{}_{4}$

Definition:

$\underline{}_{1}\ \underline{}_{2}\ \underline{}_{3}\ \underline{}_{4}\ \underline{}_{5}:\quad \underline{}_{6}\quad \underline{}_{7}\ \underline{}_{8}\ \underline{}_{9}\ \underline{}_{10}\ \underline{}_{11}$

$\underline{}_{12}\ \underline{}_{13}\ \underline{}_{14}\ \underline{}_{15}\quad \underline{}_{16}\quad \underline{}_{17}\ \underline{}_{18}\ \underline{}_{19}\ \underline{}_{20}\ \underline{}_{21}\ \underline{}_{22}$

$\underline{}_{23}\ \underline{}_{24}\ \underline{}_{25}\ \underline{}_{26}$

2. popular boat in Venice

$\overline{}\overline{}\overline{}\overline{}\overline{}\overline{}\overline{}$
8   26   18   25   21   2   5

today I think, yesterday I . . .

$\overline{}$
22   10   17   7   27   13   12

what dentures replace

9   24   3   20   23

fruit with thick yellow skin

6   11   18   4   18   14

opposite of **more**

2   19   15   28

Tiger Woods's sport

16   26   2   1

bags you take on a trip

2   7   27   16   11   8   24

Definition:

____ ____ ____ ____ :   ____   ____ ____ ____   ____ ____ ____ ____
1   2   3   4   5   6   7   8   9   10   11   12

____ ____ ____   ____ ____ ____ ____   ____ ____   ____ ____ ____
13   14   15   16   17   18   19   20   21   22   23   24

____ ____ ____ ____
25   26   27   28

3. main event at a boxing match

    11   21   17   28   19

natural fabric used in shirts

    24   2   8   20   15   22

road or avenue

    5   6   14   12   4   8

number between 50 and 100

    10   21   27   1   29   7

knitted or crocheted blanket

    25   16   23   9   13   3

nickname for **Susan**

    5   26   18

farther up

    28   21   27   1   12   14

Definition:

  1 2 3 4 5 6 7 :   8 9 10

 11 12 13 14   15 16   17 18 19 20 21 22 23

 24 25 26 27 28 29

4. elected head of a state

$\overline{13}$ $\overline{6}$ $\overline{21}$ $\overline{34}$ $\overline{26}$ $\overline{3}$ $\overline{20}$ $\overline{19}$

body part between your hip
and your knee

$\overline{31}$ $\overline{33}$ $\overline{25}$ $\overline{13}$ $\overline{10}$

spot on a radio dial

$\overline{29}$ $\overline{14}$ $\overline{2}$ $\overline{27}$ $\overline{28}$ $\overline{6}$ $\overline{30}$

American fruits

$\overline{35}$ $\overline{18}$ $\overline{36}$ $\overline{1}$ $\overline{22}$ $\overline{5}$

one-twelfth of a year

$\overline{7}$ $\overline{20}$ $\overline{12}$ $\overline{17}$ $\overline{15}$

the base of grass

$\overline{24}$ $\overline{11}$ $\overline{19}$ $\overline{9}$

an opinion given to you

$\overline{16}$ $\overline{4}$ $\overline{21}$ $\overline{28}$ $\overline{32}$ $\overline{8}$

divisions in a book

$\overline{32}$ $\overline{10}$ $\overline{16}$ $\overline{36}$ $\overline{17}$ $\overline{8}$ $\overline{26}$ $\overline{23}$

Definition:

$\overline{1}$ $\overline{2}$ $\overline{3}$ $\overline{4}$: $\overline{5}$ $\overline{6}$ $\overline{7}$ $\overline{8}$ $\overline{9}$ $\overline{10}$ $\overline{11}$ $\overline{12}$ $\overline{13}$

$\overline{14}$ $\overline{15}$ $\overline{16}$ $\overline{17}$ $\overline{18}$ $\overline{19}$ $\overline{20}$ $\overline{21}$ $\overline{22}$ $\overline{23}$

$\overline{24}$ $\overline{25}$ $\overline{26}$ $\overline{27}$ $\overline{28}$ $\overline{29}$ $\overline{30}$ $\overline{31}$, $\overline{32}$ $\overline{33}$ $\overline{34}$ $\overline{35}$ $\overline{36}$

TARGET AREA 3: Definition Usage   Building Words

*DIRECTIONS: Start with one letter and keep adding a letter to make words that fit the definitions. The letters are in the correct order for each word. See **CLUES** for help.*

1.   ___   me, myself

          ___ ___   opposite of **out**

          ___ ___ ___   be first in a race

          ___ ___ ___ ___   alcoholic drink made from grapes

          ___ ___ ___ ___ ___   strong string

---

2.   ___   letter that looks like a circle

          ___ ___   opposite of **off**

          ___ ___ ___   the first number

          ___ ___ ___ ___   condition of muscles

          ___ ___ ___ ___ ___   a pebble or small rock

---

3.   ___   first letter of alphabet

          ___ ___   similar to

          ___ ___ ___   what is left after a fire

          ___ ___ ___ ___   hair on your eyelid

          ___ ___ ___ ___ ___   sudden burst of light

Workbook for Cognitive Skills copyright © Susan Howell Brubaker 2009

4. ___   letter sounding like **pea**

    ___ ___   short name for **father**

    ___ ___ ___   average score in a golf game

    ___ ___ ___ ___   a piece of something

    ___ ___ ___ ___ ___   a celebration for a birthday

---

5. ___ ___   exist

    ___ ___ ___   make a wager

    ___ ___ ___ ___   the most excellent

    ___ ___ ___ ___ ___   a large animal

    ___ ___ ___ ___ ___ ___   turkey white meat

---

6. ___ ___   short word for **mother**

    ___ ___ ___   male adult

    ___ ___ ___ ___   central part

    ___ ___ ___ ___ ___   New England state

    ___ ___ ___ ___ ___ ___   referring to the seas

TARGET AREA 3: Definition Usage   Word Addition

DIRECTIONS: Write the word for each definition on the lines to the right. The word that is defined in bold print is composed of your three previous answers written in order. See **CLUES** *for help.*

1. myself   __ __

    in a location   __ __

    tennis, foot, or volley _____   __ __ __ __

    item to put on spaghetti

    __ __ __ __ __ __ __ __

2. spoked part of a bicycle   __ __ __ __ __

    informal place to drink   __ __ __

    use oars in a boat   __ __ __

    a cart with one wheel and two handles

    __ __ __ __ __ __ __ __ __ __ __

3. opposite of **good**   __ __ __

    after-dinner candy   __ __ __ __

    opposite of **off**   __ __

    net game played with a birdie

    __ __ __ __ __ __ __ __ __ __

4. writing utensil containing ink   ___ ___ ___

    male adult   ___ ___ ___

    another name for a boat   ___ ___ ___ ___

    quality or style of handwriting

    ___ ___ ___ ___ ___ ___ ___ ___ ___

---

5. opposite of **in**   ___ ___ ___

    man's name   ___ ___ ___ ___

    sound a small bell makes   ___ ___ ___ ___

    it describes bills that have not been paid

    ___ ___ ___ ___ ___ ___ ___ ___ ___ ___ ___

---

6. section of a school year   ___ ___ ___ ___

    opposite of **out**   ___ ___

    having already eaten   ___ ___ ___

    to end something

    ___ ___ ___ ___ ___ ___ ___ ___ ___

---

7. except for   ___ ___ ___

    2,000 pounds   ___ ___ ___

    open space in the ground   ___ ___ ___ ___

    part of the fastening on a shirt or blouse

    ___ ___ ___ ___ ___ ___ ___ ___ ___ ___

8.   not old   __ __ __

        pampering place   __ __ __

        miles ___ hour   __ __ __

source of information on current events

__ __ __ __ __ __ __ __ __

---

9.   another spelling of **two**   __ __

        short name for **advertisement**   __ __

        three-legged seat   __ __ __ __ __

type of mushroom

__ __ __ __ __ __ __ __ __

---

10.   an automobile   __ __ __

        use a shovel   __ __ __

        _____ apple; one apple   __ __

style of sweater

__ __ __ __ __ __ __ __

---

11.   man's name   __ __ __

        sandwich place   __ __ __ __

        opposite of **off**   __ __

weed with a yellow blossom

__ __ __ __ __ __ __ __ __

TARGET AREA 3: Definition Usage   Word Splits

DIRECTIONS: The longest word is described first. The letters in the next two words should be combined and rearranged to make up the first word. The blanks give you the number of letters in the words. See CLUES for help.

1. __ __ __ __ __ __ __   place where planes take off

     __ __ __ __   sound a lion makes

     __ __ __   center of a plum

2. __ __ __ __ __ __ __ __   commits or makes a vow

     __ __ __ __   heavy cord or twine

     __ __ __ __   title for a single woman

3. __ __ __ __ __ __   pal or buddy

     __ __ __   color of blood

     __ __ __   flapping part of a fish

4. __ __ __ __ __ __ __   game played for prizes

     __ __ __ __   price you pay for something

     __ __ __   two less than a dozen

5. __ __ __ __ __ __ __   gymnast

   __ __ __ __   vehicle driven on water

   __ __ __   vehicle driven on land

---

6. __ __ __ __ __ __ __ __   Christmas decoration

   __ __ __ __   strip of hair on a horse

   __ __ __ __   ripped

---

7. __ __ __ __ __ __ __   wind storm

   __ __ __ __   enter through this

   __ __ __   light brown

---

8. __ __ __ __ __   it goes with hope and charity

   __ __ __   opposite of **thin**

   __ __   short word for **hello**

---

9. __ __ __ __ __ __ __   person who is in charge

   __ __ __ __   female horse

   __ __ __   very old horse

10. __ __ __ __ __ __ __   to crash into

           __ __ __ __   Barbie or Ken toy

           __ __ __   frozen water

---

11. __ __ __ __ __ __ __ __   place with a sink and toilet

           __ __ __ __ __   use this to sweep the floor

           __ __ __   head covering

---

12. __ __ __ __ __ __   5, 47, or 466

           __ __ __   type of liquor

           __ __ __   male name

---

13. __ __ __ __ __ __ __ __   type of jewelry

           __ __ __ __ __   not fuzzy

           __ __ __   wager

---

14. __ __ __ __ __ __ __ __   type of bird kept as a pet

           __ __ __ __   fruit from a tree

           __ __ __ __   nickname for **Katherine**

TARGET AREA 3: Definition Usage   Chained Words

DIRECTIONS: *Write the answers to the first two words. When you read your answers with the letter between them, they make up the final word. A description for each missing word is given. See* **CLUES** *for help.*

1. _____ + **I** + _____ = _____
   taxi   fish snare   cupboard

2. _____ + **A** + _____ = _____
   myself   certain   use a ruler

3. _____ + **A** + _____ = _____
   large   belongs to me   having two wives

4. _____ + **A** + _____ = _____
   feline pet   piece of wood   book of items

5. _____ + **I** + _____ = _____
   a penny   rating   not Fahrenheit

6. _____ + **O** + _____ = _____
   man's nickname   piece of chain   bird

7. _____ + **O** + _____ = _____
   she   opposite of **out**   illegal drug

8. _____ + **I** + _____ = _____
   body part   thin roofing rock   make laws

9. _____ + **A** + _____ = _____
   man's name   big bird   Indian weapon

10. _____ + **I** + _____ = _____
   join together   use a knife   a state

11. _____ + **I** + _____ = _____
   damage slightly   jewelry metal   a flower

12. _____ + **O** + _____ = _____
   hotel   a penny   not guilty

13. _____ + **I** + _____ = _____
   paintings   strangle   spiny green vegetable

14. _____ + **E** + _____ = _____
   woman's name   pool stick   grill outdoors

15. _____ + **A** + _____ = _____
   pot   mother   southern country

16. _____ + **I** + _____ = _____
   insect   make ice   product for cold climates

17. _____ + **I** + _____ = _____
   opposite of **off**   opposite of **off**   vegetable

TARGET AREA 3: Definition Usage   Changing Phrases

DIRECTIONS: Start with the word in bold print and change one letter to make the word that
fits into a two-word phrase. Change one letter of that word to make the second
*word on the next line and so on. See **CLUES** for help.*

1. Start with **FAT**

tabby _____

place _____

gentle _____

tin _____

racing _____

3. Start with **WEE**

spider _____

soaking _____

fishing _____

macademia _____

absolutely _____

2. Start with **HAM**

ten-gallon _____

boiling _____

ground _____

bull _____

polka _____

4. Start with **LIE**

apple _____

safety _____

ballpoint _____

lion's _____

Cornish _____

5. | Start with **DIM** |

beaver _____

Uncle _____

jig _____

criminal _____

lock _____

8. | Start with **MOM** |

peeping _____

Tiny _____

bow _____

stubbed _____

tank _____

6. | Start with **MUD** |

coffee _____

bed _____

hooked _____

back _____

bath _____

9. | Start with **TEN** |

chamomile _____

Mediterranean _____

matching _____

teacher's _____

peach _____

7. | Start with **LOCK** |

Little _____

argyle _____

knap _____

six- _____

trailer _____

10. | Start with **ROSE** |

panty _____

button _____

totem _____

starring _____

Tootsie _____

TARGET AREA 3: Definition Usage   Rhyming Phrases

DIRECTIONS: The unusual definition gives a clue to two words that rhyme and begin with the letters shown. The words are common ones but are not usually put together to form the phrase. See CLUES for help.

1. dill that costs five cents

   n ___ ___ ___ ___ ___   **p** ___ ___ ___ ___ ___

2. large hog

   b ___ ___   **p** ___ ___

3. unhappy father

   s ___ ___   **d** ___ ___ ___

4. inexpensive animals that give us wool

   c ___ ___ ___ ___   **s** ___ ___ ___ ___

5. romantic meeting at midnight

   l ___ ___ ___   **d** ___ ___ ___ ___

6. honest-to-goodness great bargain

   r ___ ___ ___   **d** ___ ___ ___

7. top-rated visitor

   b __ __ __   **g** __ __ __ __

---

8. one of fifty wonderful divisions in America

   g __ __ __ __   **s** __ __ __ __

---

9. two unusual things that belong together

   r __ __ __   **p** __ __ __

---

10. humorous rabbit

    f __ __ __ __   **b** __ __ __ __

---

11. strange-looking hair growth on a man's face

    w __ __ __ __   **b** __ __ __ __

---

12. nice-quality lumber

    g __ __ __   **w** __ __ __

---

13. great-quality alcoholic beverage

    f __ __ __   **w** __ __ __

---

14. place for stray hunting dogs

    h __ __ __ __   **p** __ __ __ __

15. place where a headache starts and what it brings

   b __ __ __ __   **p** __ __ __

16. shop you own

   y __ __ __   **s** __ __ __ __

17. four-legged seat you do not need

   s __ __ __ __   **c** __ __ __ __

18. an ability to use a tool to bore holes

   d __ __ __ __   **s** __ __ __ __

19. furniture in which a visitor can store things

   g __ __ __ __   **c** __ __ __ __

20. sniffling and sneezing you have had for a long while

   o __ __   **c** __ __ __

21. place to store unwanted stuff

   j __ __ __   **t** __ __ __ __

22. head of the burglars

   c __ __ __ __   **t** __ __ __ __

TARGET AREA 4:
Letter Placement

TARGET AREA 4: Letter Placement   Omitted Letter

DIRECTIONS: *Omit one letter from each word to make a new word. Do this a second time but omit a different letter from the original word. See **CLUES** for help.*

1. learn   _____   _____

2. moist   _____   _____

3. booth   _____   _____

4. raid   _____   _____

5. heard   _____   _____

6. brain   _____   _____

7. dime   _____   _____

8. champ   _____   _____

9. solid   _____   _____

10. coat   _____   _____

11. yearn   _____   _____

12. plump   _____   _____

13. pare   _____   _____

14. grown _____   _____

15. smash _____   _____

16. carve _____   _____

17. weight _____   _____

18. cube _____   _____

19. stable _____   _____

20. gland _____   _____

21. pint _____   _____

22. every _____   _____

23. range _____   _____

24. breed _____   _____

25. hearth _____   _____

26. tray _____   _____

27. stack _____   _____

28. flame _____   _____

TARGET AREA 4: Letter Placement   Disguised Words

DIRECTIONS: The words in each category really do belong there. Change one letter in
each word so that you form a word that fits in the category. For example,
in question 1, slower *would become* shower. *See* **CLUES** *for help.*

1. BATHROOM ITEMS

towed _____

silk _____

scare _____

wills _____

bomb _____

snap _____

3. THINGS YOU READ

boot _____

paler _____

ward _____

nose _____

navel _____

wetter _____

2. ANIMALS

timer _____

fear _____

coat _____

loose _____

beaker _____

pull _____

sleep _____

4. FISH

grout _____

tuba _____

paddock _____

porch _____

crib _____

boss _____

share _____

5. COLORS

pine _____

tar _____

sold _____

greed _____

creak _____

grab _____

blank _____

7. CLOTHING

tin _____

best _____

press _____

rope _____

parts _____

cost _____

shots _____

6. WEATHER

fox _____

slept _____

farm _____

story _____

snob _____

ruin _____

flooring _____

kind child _____

8. THINGS WITH A POINT

jaw _____

men _____

pig _____

wart _____

swore _____

stay _____

mail _____

form _____

TARGET AREA 4: Letter Placement

*DIRECTIONS: The letters in each box are used to spell words that fit the definitions. Change the order of the letters to make three different words. See **CLUES** for help.*

1. **O P S T**

   large stick to anchor a fence   _____

   spinning toys   _____

   common name for a dalmation   _____

2. **B S T U**

   end part of a ticket   _____

   places to take baths   _____

   statue of the upper body only   _____

3. **A E M N**

   last word in a prayer   _____

   not nice; nasty   _____

   people call you by this   _____

4. **D I K S**

   small flat round object   _____

   general name for children   _____

   slide out of control when driving   _____

5. **D E I S T**

    they help you lose weight   _____

    makes changes to improve writing   _____

    high and low ocean currents   _____

6. **A C E R T**

    prepare food to bring to an affair   _____

    large wooden box with slats   _____

    copy something through thin paper   _____

7. **E E H R T**

    sometimes called "laughing gas"   _____

    opposite of **here**   _____

    the number after two   _____

8. **B E I R S U**

    black-and-blue area on a body   _____

    hides something under the ground   _____

    expensive red gems   _____

9. **A E L S T**

not fresh; like old bread   _____

take what does not belong to you   _____

opposite of **most**   _____

---

10. **A B E K R**

chef who makes pastries   _____

put your foot on it to stop a car   _____

damage something   _____

---

11. **A D E I P R S**

sadness; depression   _____

underwear for infants   _____

spoke highly of someone   _____

---

12. **A D E L P**

lost the color in your face   _____

part of a bicycle   _____

beg and beg someone   _____

13. **A E M S T**

ribs, steaks, chops, hamburger, etc. _____

hot water in misty form _____

groups of players form these in sports _____

14. **D R E A N G**

female goose _____

flower bed _____

warning of something harmful _____

15. **A P R S E**

an extra tire _____

yellowish green tree fruits _____

weapon with a sharp point _____

16. **T A L E P**

ironed or stitched fold in material _____

dish for food _____

delicate part of a flower _____

TARGET AREA 4: Letter Placement

*DIRECTIONS: Write a word to fit each definition in each of the numbered items. If you know the first definition, the second definition is the **same word** spelled backward. See **CLUES** for help.*

1. put a stopper into something   _____

    swallow loudly   _____

2. sticky black material   _____

    small rodent   _____

3. number after nine   _____

    center part of a tennis court   _____

4. shake your head in agreement   _____

    man's name   _____

5. a fight between nations   _____

    not cooked; like sushi   _____

6. eight-sided traffic sign   _____

    cooking containers   _____

7. buddies or friends

    hit someone with your hand

_____

_____

8. wild animal that looks like a dog

    go with the _____

_____

_____

9. warm and cozy

    rifles and revolvers

_____

_____

10. trade one thing for something else

    animals' feet

_____

_____

11. tiny black mammals that fly at night

    kill someone with a knife

_____

_____

12. not the whole thing

    device to capture an animal

_____

_____

13. do not give away; save

    take a quick look

_____

_____

14. a dresser compartment

    money promised if something is returned

_____

_____

TARGET AREA 4: Letter Placement

*DIRECTIONS: Each word is missing one letter. If you complete the words correctly, each letter of the alphabet will be used only **once**. See **CLUES** for help.*

A B C D E F G H I J K L M N O P Q R S T U V W X Y Z

1. A C C E ___ T

2. B A ___ A A R

3. C A S H E ___

4. D I A ___ R A M

5. E ___ E C U T I V E

6. F O R ___ A L

7. G R O ___ C H

8. H E ___ G E H O G

9. ___ N D U S T R Y

10. J O U R ___ A L

11. K N U ___ K L E

12. L A C ___ U E R

13. M A T R I M O N ___

14. N O V E ___

15. O F ___ E R

16. P R O ___ L E M

17. Q U A R ___ E R

18. R E ___ I E W

19. S U B ___ E C T

20. T I C ___ L E

21. U N L ___ S S

22. V ___ R I E T Y

23. W A L R U ___

24. X- ___ A Y

25. Y O U T ___

26. Z E R ___

A B C D E F G H I J K L M N O P Q R S T U V W X Y Z

1. AF ___ LUENT

2. BAPTI ___ E

3. CAMPAI ___ N

4. DA ___ P

5. E ___ PLOSION

6. FL ___ ID

7. GOP ___ ER

8. HEA ___ Y

9. IN ___ UIRE

10. JO ___ ING

11. K ___ EAD

12. LAW ___ ER

13. MEDI ___ AL

14. NEPHE ___

15. OB ___ ECT

16. PEL ___ CAN

17. QUAI ___

18. RAIN ___ OW

19. SCOL ___

20. TRO ___ HY

21. URG ___

22. VIC ___ ORY

23. WOR ___ E

24. XYL ___ PHONE

25. YE ___ ST

26. ZEB ___ A

A B C D E F G H I J K L M N O P Q R S T U V W X Y Z

1. AM ___ SE

2. BO ___ ER

3. CAN ___ LE

4. DI ___ TANT

5. ERR ___ ND

6. FLO ___ ERS

7. GR ___ AN

8. HAL ___

9. IN ___ ERIT

10. JE ___ SEY

11. K ___ OWN

12. LIBER ___ Y

13. MANUA ___

14. NI ___ HT

15. OAT ___ EAL

16. PRI ___ ATE

17. QUA ___ K

18. RE ___ ECT

19. S ___ UASH

20. TULI ___

21. UMP ___ RE

22. VOCA ___ ULARY

23. WI ___ ARD

24. DAIR ___

25. YAN ___ EE

26. Z ___ ST

A B C D E F G H I J K L M N O P Q R S T U V W X Y Z

1. S ___ OIL

2. HA ___ ARD

3. CURFE ___

4. ___ ENTLE

5. FO ___ ES

6. CO ___ EDY

7. VAL ___ E

8. SUE ___ E

9. MO ___ ST

10. FAVO ___

11. LOGI ___

12. ___ UILT

13. ___ IELD

14. T ___ ICK

15. CHIE ___

16. SC ___ NT

17. SMOO ___ H

18. CA ___ ITY

19. EN ___ OY

20. BUC ___ ET

21. MEM ___ ER

22. R ___ ISE

23. NERVOU ___

24. LO ___ ELY

25. B ___ ANK

26. PR ___ UD

A B C D E F G H I K L M N O P R S T U V W Y Z

1. ___ HOST

2. FLAMING ___

3. ___ RIVER

4. ___ HEATER

5. HOW ___

6. ___ GAIN

7. ___ LAKE

8. ___ ARROW

9. ___ RANCH

10. ___ QUALITY

11. ___ ALLEY

12. ___ DEAL

13. ___ LOVER

14. ___ NEATEN

15. CRATE ___

16. QUART ___

17. ___ NOT

18. FAR ___

19. ___ AWNING

20. ___ RICE

21. ___ HEEL

22. HEART ___

23. ___ HAVE

TARGET AREA 4: Letter Placement   Repeated Letters

DIRECTIONS: *Insert the same letter multiple times into the blanks by each number to make a word. Some letters are used more than once and not all letters are used. See **CLUES** for help.*

A B C D E F G H I J K L M N O P Q R S T U V W X Y Z

1. __ I __ T H   13. E L E __ T R I __

2. __ H A __ I   14. P __ R __ D E

3. __ C __ N G   15. F __ A N N E __

4. __ A D A __   16. M __ T __ R

5. __ A F F O __ I L   17. A N __ B O D __

6. S U __ U R __ A N   18. __ I P __ O E

7. __ E A D A C __ E   19. D I __ A __ T E R

8. M O R __ I __ G   20. __ A R B A __ E

9. H __ M O R O __ S   21. __ E O __ L E

10. F __ E E Z E __   22. __ I N D O __

11. __ E R O __   23. B R __ A T H __

12. __ E L __ E T

Continue as directed on page 194 and use the same letter twice in each word.

A B C D E F G H I J K L M N O P Q R S T U V W X Y Z

1. A ___ ___ RACTIVE

2. PION ___ ___ R

3. QUA ___ ___ EL

4. ETIQUE ___ ___ E

5. MI ___ ___ LE

6. GO ___ ___ IP

7. MATIN ___ ___

8. JI ___ ___ LE

9. MA ___ ___ EQUIN

10. SCRI ___ ___ LE

11. HAWA ___ ___ AN

12. BA ___ ___ ERINA

13. SW ___ ___ T

14. CAB ___ ___ SE

15. HI ___ ___ UPS

16. DANDRU ___ ___

17. LA ___ ___ ER

18. FIS ___ ___ OOK

19. PI ___ ___ A

20. TOBA ___ ___ O

21. FO ___ ___ IL

22. HA ___ ___ INESS

23. ZU ___ ___ HINI

24. A ___ ___ ONIA

25. VAC ___ ___ M

26. I ___ ___ ATURE

Workbook for Cognitive Skills copyright © Susan Howell Brubaker 2009

Continue as directed on page 194 but insert three of the same letter.

A B C D E F G H I J K L M N O P Q R S T U V W X Y Z

1. DRE ___ ___ E ___

2. ART ___ F ___ C ___ AL

3. ___ E ___ ___ ERMINT

4. A ___ TE ___ ___ A

5. ___ U ___ ___ LES

6. ___ REA ___ MEN ___

7. PO ___ ___ O ___

8. ___ E ___ ICATE ___

9. SU ___ ___ ENDE ___

10. E ___ ___ NO ___

11. A ___ ___ EMP ___

12. B ___ LI ___ V ___

13. ___ UM ___ LE ___ EE

14. ___ AXI ___ U ___

15. C ___ N ___ D ___

16. SN ___ ___ Z ___

17. PARA ___ ___ E ___

18. ___ O ___ KROA ___ H

19. ___ IVI ___ E ___

20. ___ IG ___ LIG ___ T

21. C ___ RP ___ RATI ___ N

22. ___ DV ___ NT ___ GE

23. U ___ DERSTA ___ DI ___ G

24. ___ N ___ S ___ AL

25. ___ LU ___ ___ Y

26. HO ___ TE ___ ___

27. ___ INEA ___ ___ LE

28. B ___ K ___ N ___

29. MI ___ ___ O ___

30. C ___ C ___ ___ N

TARGET AREA 4: Letter Placement   Multiple Missing Letters

DIRECTIONS: Write a letter on each blank to complete the words. If you complete the words correctly, each letter of the alphabet will be used just once. See **CLUES** *for help.*

A B C D E F G H I J K L M N O P Q R S T U V W X Y Z

1. ___ ard ___ are

2. ___ om ___ ort

3. ___ itche ___

4. forei ___ n

5. la ___ ender

6. ___ eyon ___

7. si ___ teen

8. nu ___ ser ___

9. mas ___ uerad ___

10. c ___ nna ___ on

11. ___ ainter

12. ___ b ___ ective

13. ___ o ___ dier

14. cra ___ y

15. lea ___ her

16. pe ___ n ___ t

A B C D E F G H I J K L M N O P Q R S T U V W X Y Z

1. c ___ co ___ ut

2. ___ eaknes ___

3. or ___ hid

4. stan ___ a ___ d

5. in ___ ury

6. ___ ualif ___

7. ___ raph

8. ___ us ___ and

9. e ___ otic

10. h ___ mmoc ___

11. ___ eas ___ oon

12. un ___ ___ orm

13. lea ___ es

14. bla ___ er

15. w ___ lco ___ e

16. cr ___ mb ___ e

Workbook for Cognitive Skills copyright © Susan Howell Brubaker 2009

A B C D E F G H I J K L M N O P Q R S T U V W X Y Z

1. wed ___ e

2. ___ romot ___ on

3. ___ ogging

4. ___ ight ___ are

5. un ___ app ___

6. e ___ uat ___ r

7. do ___ en

8. lob ___ te ___

9. oli ___ es

10. e ___ hale

11. in ___ la ___ ion

12. bas ___ ___ t

13. gro ___ l

14. m ___ star ___

15. su ___ stan ___ e

16. fin ___ ___ ly

A B C D E F G H I J K L M N O P Q R S T U V W X Y Z

1. a ___ ult

2. ___ re ___ kles

3. fo ___ e ___ er

4. li ___ rar ___

5. ___ uic ___ ly

6. pr ___ v ___ ew

7. an ___ ie ___ y

8. ___ a ___ ority

9. ima ___ i ___ e

10. p ___ y ___ ical

11. b ___ llot

12. l ___ ke ___ arm

13. mu ___ ti ___ ly

14. ap ___ logi ___ e

TARGET AREA 4: Letter Placement

*DIRECTIONS: In each group, use only the letters in the box to fill in the blanks in each word. The letters can be in any order. See **CLUES** for help.*

A B C

___ ___ b ___ age

f ___ ___ ri ___

___ ___ du ___ t

___ ___ ___ k

B C D

a ___ un ___ an ___ e

___ u ___ kle ___

___ up ___ oar ___

___ raw ___ a ___ k

C D E

___ ___ u ___ ation

sli ___ ___ ___

___ o ___ ___

___ ___ ___ ay

D E F

___ e ___ ___ nd

gol ___ ___ ___

e ___ i ___ ic ___

___ ol ___ ___ r

E F G

___ or ___ ___ t

___ i ___ ht ___ r

___ ri ___ ___

r ___ ___ ri ___ erator

G H I

sl ___ ___ ___ t

clot ___ ___ n ___

we ___ ___ ___

___ ___ n ___ e

L M N

___ e ___ ta ___

___ o ___ eso ___ e

___ or ___ a ___

a ___ ___ o ___ d

M N O

c ___ ___ fir ___

___ ___ ___ ey

___ ___ ve ___ ber

___ r ___ a ___ ent

N O P

cham ___ i ___ ___

ca ___ ___ ___ y

u ___ ___ ___ ened

___ ia ___ ___

R S T

___ ___ ___ ange

te ___ mi ___ e ___

d ___ a ___ ___ ic

in ___ e ___ e ___ ting

S T U

d ___ ___ ___

as ___ a ___ l ___

man ___ ___ crip ___

h ___ ___ ___ le

T U V

c ___ lti ___ a ___ e

s ___ ppor ___ i ___ e

e ___ al ___ a ___ e

___ a ___ l ___

TARGET AREA 4: Letter Placement   Words in Words

*DIRECTIONS: Use the letters from the word on the right to fill in the blanks on the left to form a word. The letters will need to be rearranged to make a word. See **CLUES** for help.*

1. ___ cc ___ ___ ___ ance   tape

2. ___ ___ dsp ___ e ___ d   bear

3. ___ a ___ mon ___ ___ a   rich

4. kin ___ ___ ___ ___ s   send

5. ___ ed ___ ___ at ___   time

6. ___ at ___ rp ___ lla ___   rice

7. ___ ___ ___ ec ___ ally   pies

8. d ___ a ___ br ___ dg ___   wire

9. fo ___ ___ u ___ at ___   rent

10. li ___ ___ gu ___ r ___   fade

11. j ___ o ___ a ___ d ___   prey

12. ne ___ ___ p ___ ___ er   wasp

13. o ___ t ___ ___ an ___ ing   dust

14. ___ ___ a ___ a ___ tee   rung

15. ___ ___ ra ___ yz ___   leap

16. r ___ c ___ ___ n ___ le   gate

17. in ___ ___ r ___ ___ pt   true

18. qu ___ c ___ ___ an ___   kids

19. sy ___ ___ ___ theti ___   camp

20. ___ e ___ ___ gr ___ m   tale

21. ___ as ___ ion ___ b ___ e   half

22. v ___ ___ ___ an ___   cool

23. w ___ ___ d ___ ob ___   rare

TARGET AREA 4: Letter Placement   Double Insertions

*DIRECTIONS: Make a word by inserting each letter in parentheses twice. In other words, four blanks in the word should be filled with two of each letter in parentheses. See **CLUES** for help.*

1. ___ m ___ ___ a ___ e   (**i, t**)

2. ___ h ___ ___ k ___ rs   (**c, e**)

3. ___ b ___ ___ do ___   (**a, n**)

4. f ___ ___ ___ ___ w   (**l, o**)

5. ___ a ___ ___ e ___   (**b, r**)

6. ___ ___ ___ icat ___   (**d, e**)

7. ___ ___ rb ___ ___ e   (**a, g**)

8. ___ an ___ ___ or ___   (**d, l**)

9. im ___ ___ o ___ e ___   (**p, r**)

10. m ___ ___ ___ ___ le   (**i, s**)

11. qu ___ ___ a ___ i ___ n   (**o, t**)

12. s ___ a ___ ___ o ___   (**l, w**)

13. o ___ ___ ___ c ___ al   (**f, i**)

14. ___ ___ nds ___ g ___ t   (**h, i**)

Workbook for Cognitive Skills copyright © Susan Howell Brubaker 2009

15. ___ ___ ___ ste ___   (**o, r**)

16. ___ ___ il ___ o ___ d   (**a, r**)

17. ___ an ___ ___ oo ___   (**b, k**)

18. ___ i ___ t ___ ___ n   (**e, f**)

19. ___ e ___ a ___ ___   (**n, t**)

20. ha ___ ___ ine ___ ___   (**p, s**)

21. ___ o ___ the ___ ___   (**n, r**)

22. ___ ___ oug ___ ___   (**h, t**)

23. ___ ___ ___ ac ___ ous   (**i, v**)

24. a ___ c ___ h ___ ___   (**l, o**)

25. ___ n ___ aith ___ ___ l   (**f, u**)

26. po ___ ___ t ___ ca ___   (**i, l**)

27. ___ lu ___ ___ i ___ h   (**g, s**)

28. zu ___ ___ h ___ n ___   (**c, i**)

29. ___ ___ ac ___ o ___   (**r, t**)

30. ___ ___ st ___ rda ___   (**e, y**)

TARGET AREA 4: Letter Placement

Letter Pairs

DIRECTIONS: Each letter pair on the right fits twice into a word on the left. Write the letter pair two times in order to complete that word. See **CLUES** *for help.*

1. c ___ ___ rage ___ ___ s   fa

   ___ ___ iloso ___ ___ er   re

   al ___ ___ l ___ ___   ou

   t ___ ___ asu ___ ___   ma

   ___ ___ m ___ ___ l   ph

---

2. d ___ ___ gu ___ ___ e   he

   no ___ ___ e ___ ___ e   ta

   ___ ___ adac ___ ___   ic

   ___ ___ ffe ___ ___   ns

   p ___ ___ n ___ ___   is

3. ___ ___ r ___ ___ ise   ur

     ___ ___ cur ___ ___ y   po

     ___ ___ r ___ ___ lade   ac

     f ___ ___ nit ___ ___ e   ba

     p ___ ___ o ___ ___ ty   ma

     ___ ___ re ___ ___ ck   ri

---

4. ___ ___ u ___ ___ ge   em

     ___ ___ bl ___ ___   sa

     beg ___ ___ n ___ ___ g   or

     ___ ___ gib ___ ___   in

     h ___ ___ r ___ ___   po

     ___ ___ st ___ ___ ne   le

---

5. oi ___ ___ me ___ ___   ra

     l ___ ___ or ___ ___ e   ic

     a ___ ___ or ___ ___   es

     al ___ ___ in ___ ___   bs

     r ___ ___ tl ___ ___ s   nt

     f ___ ___ g ___ ___ nce   um

TARGET AREA 4: Letter Placement Word Transformation

DIRECTIONS: *The directions to this exercise are self-explanatory. Follow them carefully on each line. See CLUES for help.*

1. Print the word **PAPER** on the line below.

   _____

   In the word you wrote, change the first **P** to an **M** and the second **P** to an **N**. Write the letters on the line.

   _____

   Change the **R** to the last letter in the word **PAY**. Write the letters.

   _____

   Change the second letter to an **O**. Write the new word you formed.

   _____

---

2. Print the word **PIANO** on the line below.

   _____

   Put an **R** before the **I**. Rewrite the letters on the line.

   _____

   Switch the places of the first and last letters. Write the letters.

   _____

   Change the **I** to a **G** and drop the **P**. Write the new word you formed.

   _____

3. Print the word **CHOCOLATE** on the line.

_____

Change the first and second **O**s to an **E** and drop the **E** at the end of the word. Rewrite the letters.

_____

Exchange the places of the first two letters. Exchange the places of the fifth and sixth letters. Rewrite the letters.

_____

Replace the **H** and the **L** with the next letter of the alphabet for both of them. Rewrite the letters.

_____

Move the fifth letter to the end of the word. Replace the fifth letter with an **R**. Rewrite the letters and put a space to form two words that are associated with chocolate.

_____

4. Print the word **PEACH** on the line.

_____

Switch the places of the **P** and the **A**. Write the letters on the line.

_____

Switch the places of the second and the last letters. Write the letters.

_____

Change the second letter so it is the same as the third letter and change the fourth letter to an **L**. Write the new word you formed.

_____

TARGET AREA 4: Letter Placement

*DIRECTIONS: Next to each long box is a definition for a word that fits, using one letter per box. The lines between boxes indicate that the letter in both boxes is the same. Work back and forth between the letters and definitions to figure out the words. See **CLUES** for help.*

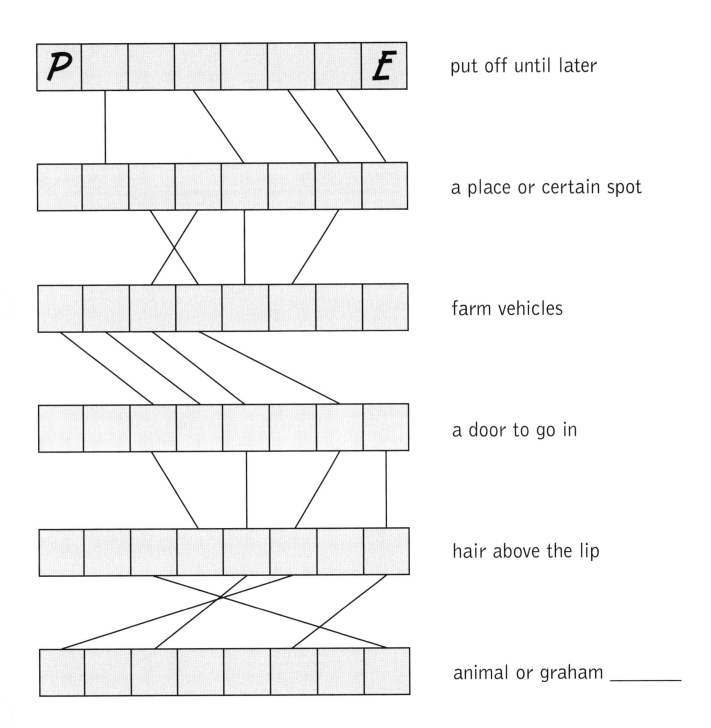

put off until later

a place or certain spot

farm vehicles

a door to go in

hair above the lip

animal or graham _____

Start with a new word and continue as on the previous page.

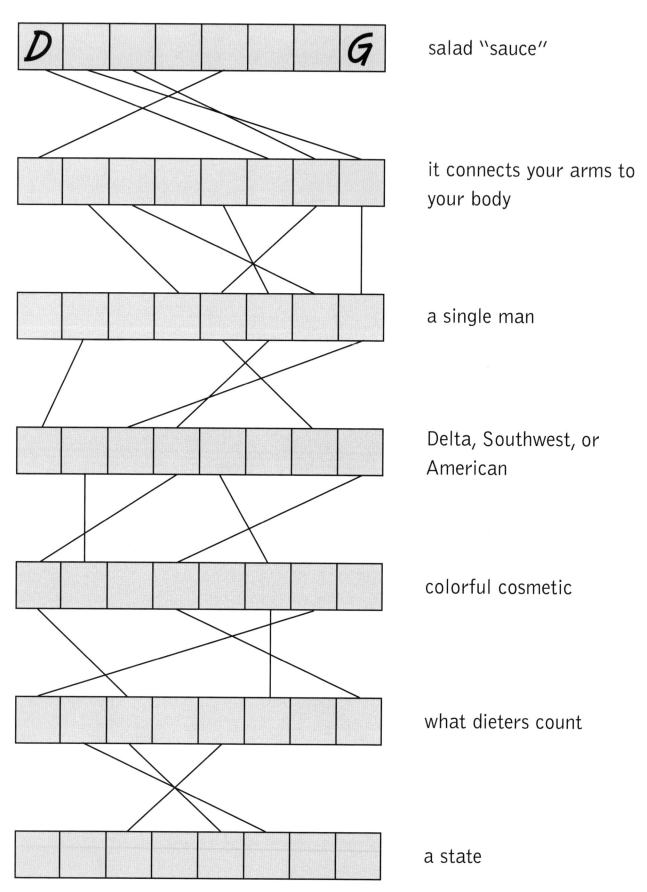

salad "sauce"

it connects your arms to your body

a single man

Delta, Southwest, or American

colorful cosmetic

what dieters count

a state

TARGET AREA 4: Letter Placement   Word Rebuses

DIRECTIONS: Add and subtract letters to each word as indicated. If you have answered correctly, a proverb will be formed reading down. See **CLUES** *for help.*

1. magnet – get + y =   _____

   that + minds – mitt =   _____

   smack + hope – chops =   _____

   lime + ghost – some =   _____

   two + bark – bat =   _____

---

2. lost + oak + in – stain =   _____

   bean + formal + pie – aim – plan =   _____

   stay + nod – stand + glue – leg =   _____

   mule + chap – much =   _____

Continue as before. This page starts a new proverb reading down.

3. bother + dye − body =   _____

lie + save − leave =   _____

most + real − last =   _____

three + fans − frees =   _____

room + new − worm =   _____

wasp + toy − tops =   _____

neat + hold − handle =   _____

mask + thin − math =   _____

cream + al − calmer =   _____

cop + water − power =   _____

TARGET AREA 4: Letter Placement

*DIRECTIONS: Choose which words will fit in the grids so that words will read across and down. Choose one word from each line. See **CLUES** for help.*

ACROSS

1. cars, bars, show

2. edit, exit, tool

3. hoot, also, else

4. seem, lean, sold

DOWN

1. deep, bees, feet

2. axle, load, sale

3. rust, list, rise

4. stem, seam, slim

    1. 2. 3. 4.

1.				
2.				
3.				
4.				

ACROSS

1. step, ship, star
2. cage, tags, hare
3. axes, able, apes
4. boot, best, born

DOWN

1. scab, skys, scam
2. tape, pear, huge
3. open, even, ages
4. neat, rest, nest

	1.	2.	3.	4.
1.				
2.				
3.				
4.				

ACROSS

1. warn, cord, word
2. idea, dean, idol
3. Rome, roam, room
4. errs, eras, bars

DOWN

1. wire, tore, care
2. idle, door, odor
3. read, rear, rake
4. dams, days, done

	1.	2.	3.	4.
1.				
2.				
3.				
4.				

TARGET AREA 4: Letter Placement   Word Alterations

DIRECTIONS: Start with the word on the left. Use the directions at the top of each column to change the original word to four new words. There are several possible answers.

	remove a letter	add a letter	change two letters	change letter order
PANS				
BEAR				
TALE				
SPIN				
MANE				
FIST				
SPEAR				
RANGE				

TARGET AREA 4: Letter Placement

Letter Fill-Ins

*DIRECTIONS: The crossword grids are incomplete. Fill in the missing letters to make words reading across and down. The letters to use are listed under the grid; however, there may be other possible solutions. Cover them unless you need the letters to complete the puzzle. See **CLUES** for help.*

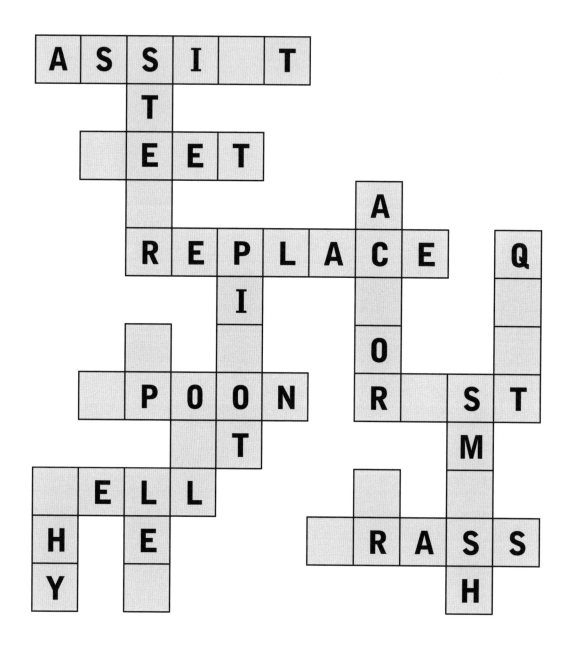

LETTERS: A E I I O U U U

D F G L S S T W

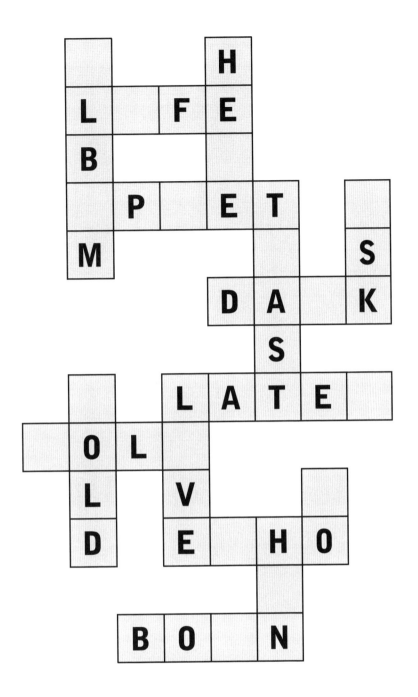

LETTERS: A A E I O O U
C F G R R R R S S

Add the vowels to complete this word puzzle. See **CLUES** *for more help.*

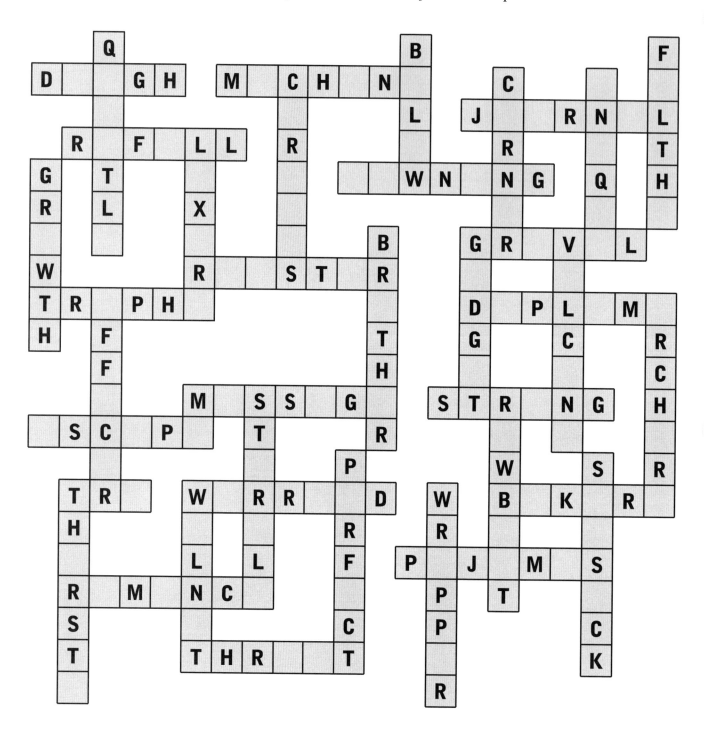

Add these letters as many times as needed to make words:

A E I O U Y

Fill in the missing letters to make words. See **CLUES** *for more help.*

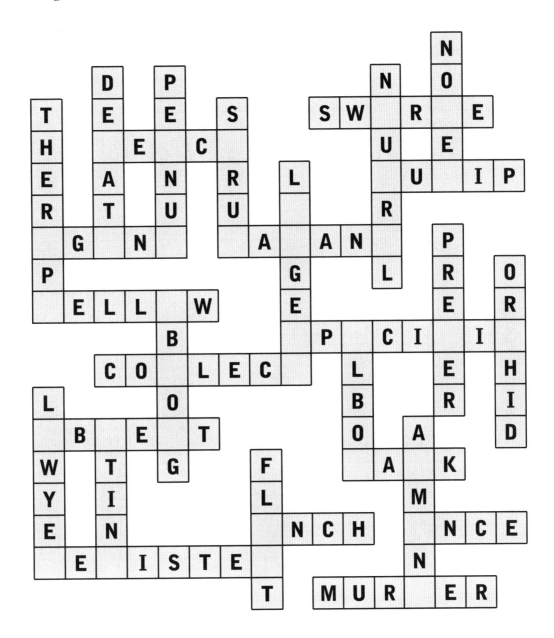

Below are the letters needed for the words. Cover them unless you need them to complete the puzzle. See CLUES for more help.

A A A A B B C D E E E F G H I L L L N N
O O O R R S S T T T V W Y

Fill in the missing letters to make words. See **CLUES** *for more help.*

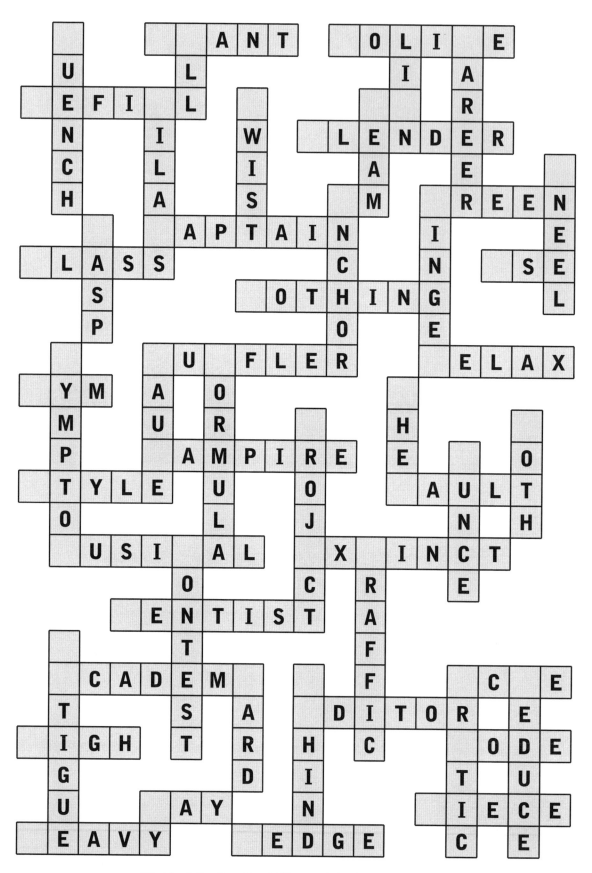

TARGET AREA 5:
Visual Logic

TARGET AREA 5: Visual Logic   Missing Elements

*DIRECTIONS: Each picture is missing one part. Write what is missing under the picture or draw in the missing element. See **CLUES** for help.*

1. _____

2. _____

3. _____

4. _____

5. _____

6. _____

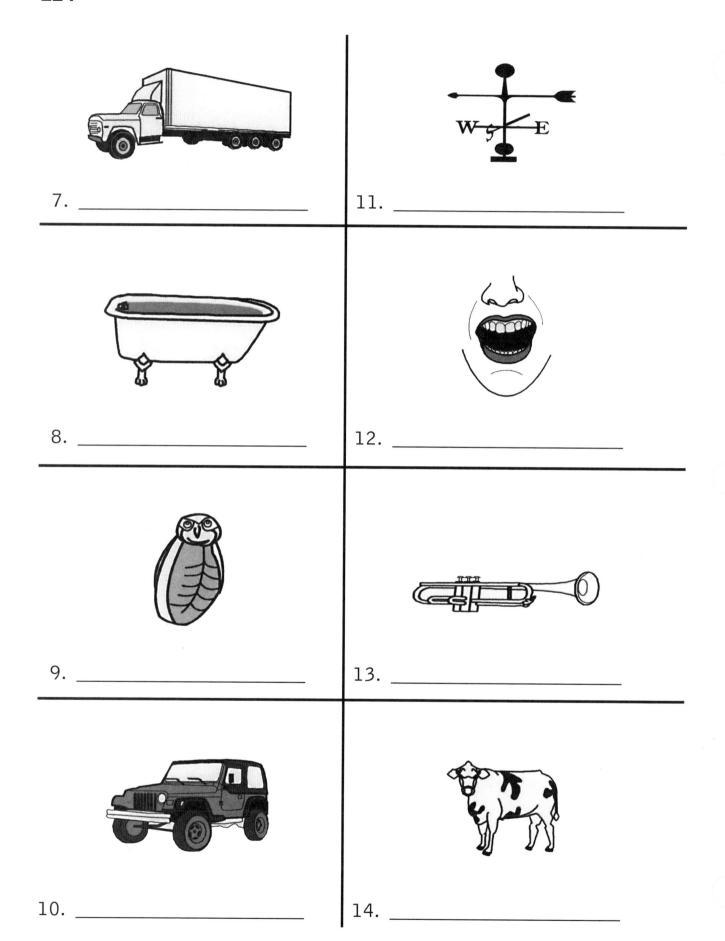

7. _____

11. _____

8. _____

12. _____

9. _____

13. _____

10. _____

14. _____

TARGET AREA 5: Visual Logic   Picture Descriptions

DIRECTIONS: Decide which picture goes with each clue. Write the number of the picture on the line next to its description. Each picture should only be used once. See CLUES for help.

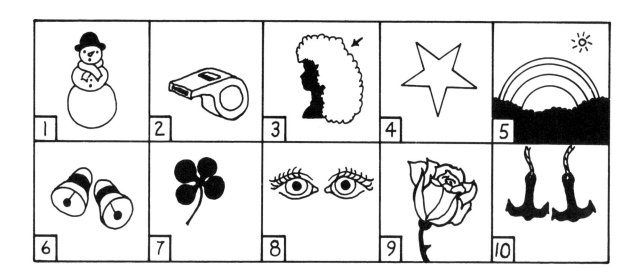

1. It has leaves. _____

2. It is the only striped object. _____

3. It is associated with a pot of gold. _____

4. You would not find the real thing in Hawaii. _____

5. The actual item would be all green in color. _____

6. It is the middle picture in the top row. _____

7. It is directly below the third answer. _____

8. If the pictures were alphabetized, it would be last on the list. _____

9. It has five points on it. _____

10. There is no description for the item in this box. _____

DIRECTIONS: *Continue as before, but notice that the titles on this page are of books, plays, and movies.*

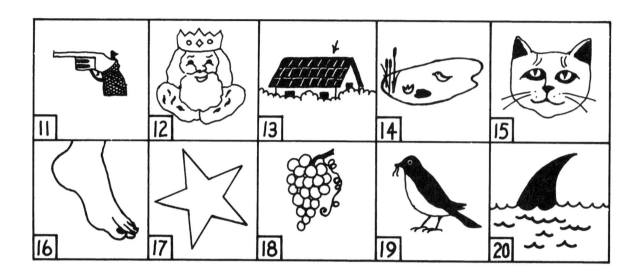

11. It grows whiskers but could not grow a beard. _____

12. It has whiskers and a beard. _____

13. It has two eyes, but you only see one in the picture. _____

14. This picture also appears on the previous page. _____

15. The picture suggests saltwater. _____

16. This picture is directly above the one in question 13. _____

17. Pictures 12, 15, and 19 have something in common with this picture. _____

18. It is manufactured (man-made). _____

19. It is associated with wine. _____

20. The box is located between the answers to questions 12 and 16. _____

DIRECTIONS: Continue as before, but notice that the items on this page are familiar phrases.

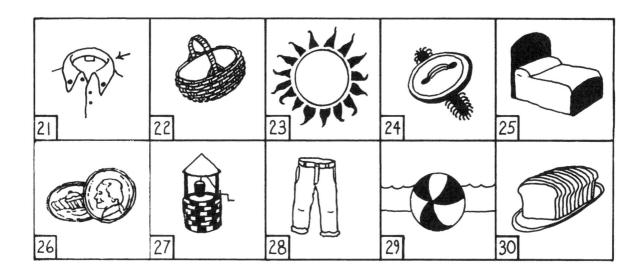

21. It is chewy. ____

22. It has a handle. ____

23. It has a zipper. ____

24. It is round in shape. ____

25. See question 29. ____

26. It has a label you can see. ____

27. It is surrounded by the answers to numbers 21, 24, and 30. ____

28. You cannot touch it. ____

29. Make a wish in this item and toss in the answer to number 25. ____

30. It is full of air. ____

TARGET AREA 5: Visual Logic

Visual Compounds

DIRECTIONS: The word for a picture on the left combined with the word for a picture on the right will form a compound word. Use each picture one time. Write the new word on the line. See **CLUES** for help.

1. _____

2. _____

3. _____

4. _____

5. _____

6. _____

7. _____

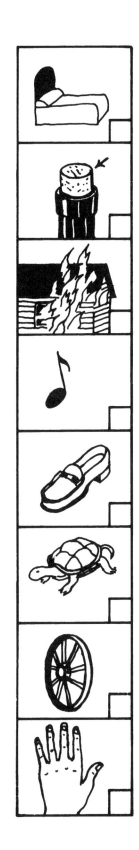

1. _____

2. _____

3. _____

4. _____

5. _____

6. _____

7. _____

8. _____

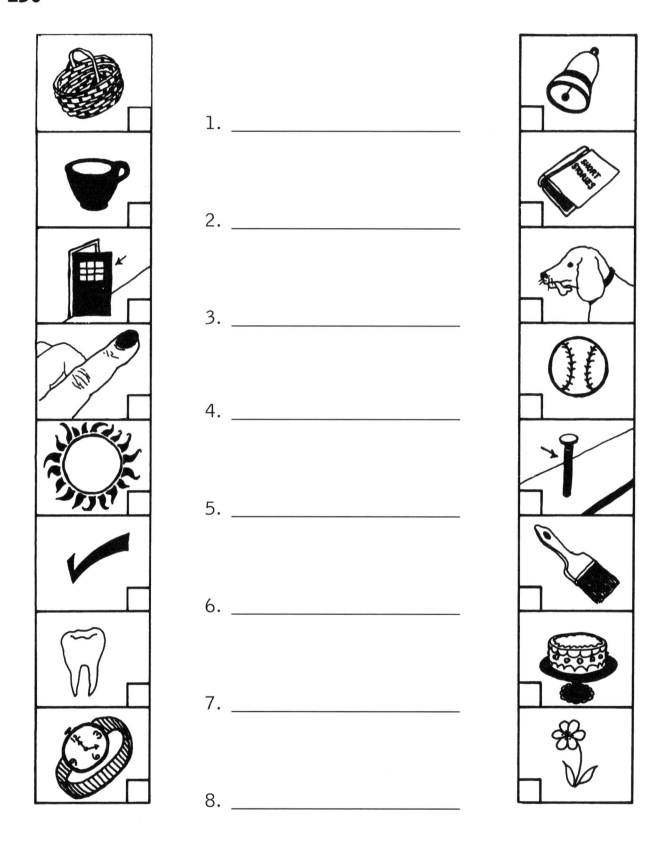

1. _____

2. _____

3. _____

4. _____

5. _____

6. _____

7. _____

8. _____

TARGET AREA 5: Visual Logic   Picture Elimination

*DIRECTIONS: Only one of the numbered pictures fits the description. Use the information to
figure out the answer and write it on the line. See **CLUES** for help.*

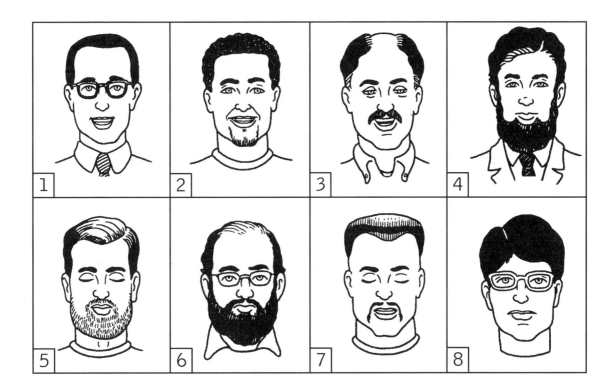

You are looking for a man who has his eyes open.

He has some hair growth on his face.

He has a full beard.

He is not wearing a suit.

The man is number _____

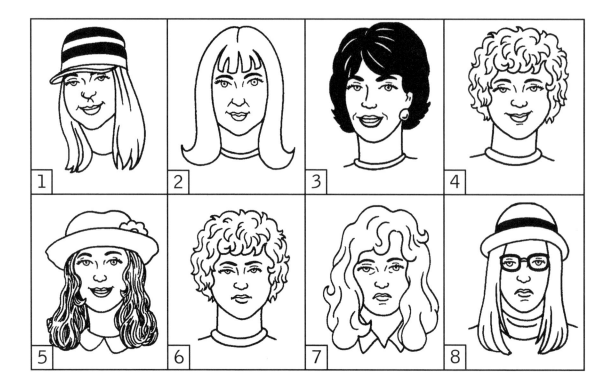

You are looking for a woman who is not wearing earrings.

She does not have short hair.

She does not have straight hair.

She is not wearing a T-shirt.

She is wearing a hat.

The woman is number _____

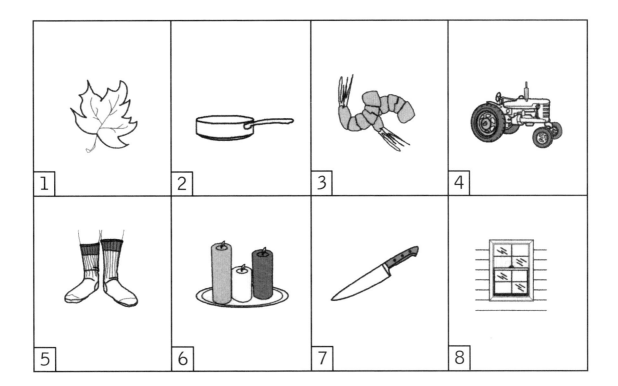

The answer item does not grow.

It would not be kept in a kitchen.

It does not feel soft.

You could not hold it in your hand.

It is not part of a house.

What is it? _____

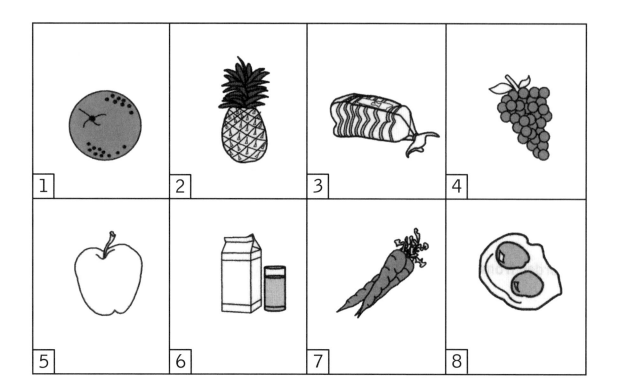

The item you are looking for can be cut into pieces.

It is a naturally growing food.

It is grown on a tree.

You would not want to chew its skin.

The answer is the easier one to peel.

What is it? _____

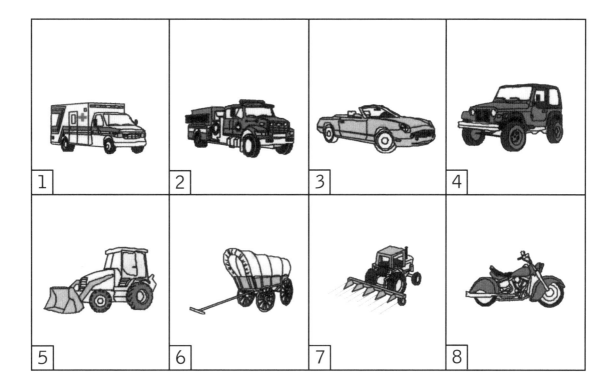

The answer is a vehicle with four wheels and a motor.

It would not fit in a normal garage.

It can carry more than two people.

The answer is the vehicle that is longer in length.

What is it? _____

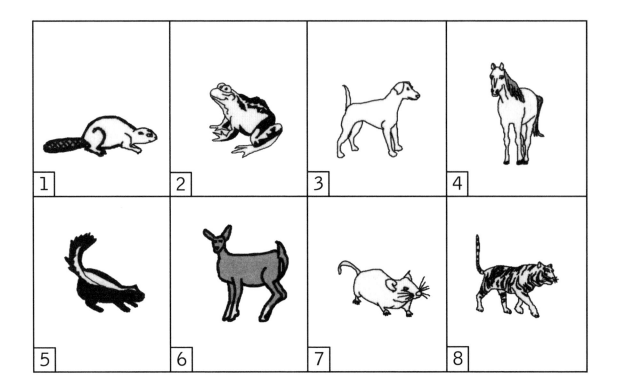

The animal you are looking for has a tail.

It does not have stripes.

It is not the smallest of the remaining animals.

It is not the slowest animal left.

It does not have hooves.

What is it? _____

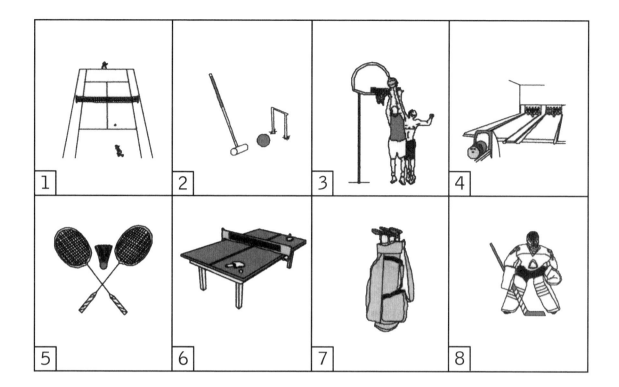

The pictures each represent a sport.

The answer sport uses some sort of ball.

The ball is hit with something in this sport.

A net is not needed to play this.

The answer is the sport that requires the least amount of space to play.

What is it? _____

TARGET AREA 5: Visual Logic   Letters in Common

DIRECTIONS: *The four words across each line share one letter. Write that letter on the line. If you have the correct letters, it will spell a place reading down. See* **CLUES** *for help.*

1. academy   brunch   civil   socks   ____

   molasses   pain   ajar   quota   ____

   bedspread   envelope   leopard   soup   ____

   survey   vertical   battery   fellow   ____

   flicker   impact   shocking   research   ____

   symbol   money   violence   action   ____

   knowledge   remedy   kidding   stopped   ____

2. charmed   washing   think   phone   ____

   account   slogan   forty   precious   ____

   puddle   detour   equal   skull   ____

   necessary   broadcast   listening   distance   ____

   predict   bottom   nothing   motto   ____

   important   equator   owner   abolish   ____

   youngster   traction   sandwich   personal   ____

3. canopy	property	burlap	episode	____
farmer	kerosene	quart	theater	____
decision	location	jockey	generous	____
avalanche	harvest	relieved	moving	____
iceberg	satin	village	noise	____
kidnap	weekend	obedient	fiddle	____
uncle	genius	harness	yeast	____
business	encourage	tonight	limestone	____
raincoat	fragrance	logic	scholar	____
miniature	ourselves	dungeon	kindergarten	____

4. parsley	banish	risk	loose	____
vacation	raising	details	advance	____
honors	nasty	winter	pecans	____
widen	liquid	created	middle	____
tapioca	claim	spirit	pillow	____
minute	violent	minister	have	____
jagged	strange	guilty	English	____
ebony	action	inventor	occupy	____

TARGET AREA 5: Visual Logic   Spoonerisms

DIRECTIONS: *Spoonerisms are made by switching the first one or two letters in a word with those of another word so that new words are made. Match a spoonerism from a choice in the first column to one in the second column. Write its number on the line. See* **CLUES** *for help.*

faded sheet _____   1. fly drag

big wallet _____   2. lamp stock

take cart _____   3. catch mats

chest base _____   4. shaded feet

miner deal _____   5. sly mice

dry flag _____   6. best chase

get moose _____   7. cake tart

stamp lock _____   8. wig ballet

match cats _____   9. met goose

my slice _____   10. diner meal

tot scale ____   1. real sting

steal ring ____   2. Scot tale

rear clock ____   3. sunny beat

sand lake ____   4. smart pile

part smile ____   5. stay gruff

gray stuff ____   6. clear rock

bunny seat ____   7. main spoon

deep shock ____   8. land sake

bare room ____   9. sheep dock

Spain moon ____   10. rare boom

---

change street ____   1. tan fool

sticky trick ____   2. hermit paste

gray train ____   3. tricky stick

chin tip ____   4. strange cheat

fan tool ____   5. belly jeans

jelly beans ____   6. dame luck

main rat ____   7. tray grain

lame duck ____   8. rain mat

permit haste ____   9. tin chip

parrot cart ____   10. carrot part

TARGET AREA 5: Visual Logic   Letter Logic

*DIRECTIONS: Read the description and write the correct letter on the line. The letters should spell a word reading down. See **CLUES** for help.*

1. The first letter is in **golf** but not in **goof**.   _____

   The second letter is in **vast** but not in **vest**.   _____

   The third letter is in **bow** but not in **boy**.   _____

   The fourth letter is in **enact** but not in **exact**.   _____

   What is the word? _____

---

2. The first letter is in **fuel** but not in **full**.   _____

   The second letter is in **own** but not in **owed**.   _____

   The third letter is in **pact** but not in **place**.   _____

   The fourth letter is in **rice** but not in **race**.   _____

   The fifth letter is in **score** but not in **scope**.   _____

   The sixth letter is in **none** but not in **no**.   _____

   What is the word? _____

3. The first letter is in **great** but not in **tear**. _____

 The second letter is in **wren** but not in **new**. _____

 The third letter is in **broader** but not in **border**. _____

 The fourth letter is in **vanilla** but not in **nail**. _____

 The fifth letter is in **invest** but not in **vents**. _____

 The sixth letter is in **task** but not in **sack**. _____

 The seventh letter is in **yield** but not in **lied**. _____

 What is the word? _____

---

4. The first letter is in **peach** but not in **ache**. _____

 The second letter is in **proper** but not in **prop**. _____

 The third letter is in **scare** but not in **sear**. _____

 The fourth letter is in **though** but not in **throng**. _____

 The fifth letter is in **smaller** but not in **steamer**. _____

 The sixth letter is in **service** but not in **scarves**. _____

 The seventh letter is in **molasses** but not in **moles**. _____

 The eighth letter is in **remark** but not in **make**. _____

 What is the word? _____

TARGET AREA 5: Visual Logic   Word Characteristics

*DIRECTIONS: Read the description and choose a word from the word list that fits it. Write the word on the line. Each word is used once. See **CLUES** for help.*

WORD LIST

SPIED	EDUCATION	GIGGLE
CARAVAN	TARTAR	CARPENTRY
UNUSUAL	DANDELION	PEELS
TENNESSEE	KNOWLEDGE	FUNGUS
STRANGEST	MADAM	BOOKKEEPER

1. It has three **G**'s in it. _____

2. It spells a different word reading backward. _____

3. The first, third, and fifth letters of the word are the same.

   _____

4. It is made of two words meaning **a good time + a man's name**.

   _____

5. It has six different consonants in it. _____

6. It contains two of each: **N**, **S**, and **E**. _____

7. If you remove the first and last letters, the word remaining is something sweet to eat. _____

8. It is made of two means of transportation with the letter **A** between them. _____

9. The last four letters spell the name of an animal. _____

10. It contains every vowel except **Y**. _____

11. It can be broken into three three-letter words, one right after the other.

    _____

12. It contains three different double letters in a row. _____

13. It is the same spelled backward or forward. _____

14. It begins and ends with the same two-letter combination.

    _____

15. It is made of a three-letter word that is repeated.

    _____

TARGET AREA 5: Visual Logic   Multiple Errors

DIRECTIONS: Below is a calendar. When you study it, you will notice that it contains many mistakes. Circle each mistake as you find it. See **CLUES** *for help.*

2007	NOVEMVER				2012	
MONDAY	**TUESDAY**	**WED.**	**THURS.**	**FRIDAY.**	**SAT.**	**SUNDAY**
					1 Teacher conf. at school 2:00 pm	**2**
3	**4** Election Day	**5**	**6**	**7**	**8** Dad's birthday	**9**
10 Pick up car at dealer	**11**	**12**	**13** Take car to dealer for new brakes	**14**	**16**	**15**
17	**18** Dad's Surprise birthday party	**19**	**20**	**21**	**22**	**23**
24 haircut- Mary 11 pm	**25**	**26**	**27** Christmas Eve	**28** Thanksgiving	**29**	**30**

Continue and circle all the mistakes or items that are not logical in the menus.

LUNCHEON MENU

SAND WITCHES

Hamburger—⅓ ounce with lettuce & tomato $4.95
   with cheese—American, Swiss, or Italian ....$.50 less
Ham and Cheese—on rye, pumperpenny, or white bread $39.95
BLT—traditional crab, lettuce, and tomato $4.95
Stacked Roast Beef—with mayo or caramel sauce $4.95

SIDE ORDERS

French Fries $2.00
Onion Triangles $2.00
Cold Slaw $2.00
Tossed Salad—choice of mustard or ketchup dressings $2.00

BEVERAGES

Coffee—regular or caffeinated $1.25
Soft Drinks—Coke, Pepsi, 8-Up, Diet Sprite, Diet Popsi $1.75
Milk—whole, skim, butter or yogurt $0.50

DINNER MENU

APPETIZERS

Beef Wings $5.50
Fresh Fruit Soup $5.25
Stufffed Mushrooms $1.25
Banana Skins with Cheese and Bacon (sour cream on request) $5.75

ENTREES

Fish and Chips with Lasagna $19.62
Stuffed Breast of Chicken with Ice Cream Sauce $10.00
New York Strip Stake—well done only $17.00
Roast Prime Rib of Beef Au Jus $18.00
Spaghetti with celery or Meetbawls $5.00
Jumbo Battered Shrimp with Special Sauce $12.01

All Entrees served with: rolls and butter, baked salad with choice of dressings, and choice
of rice (baked, fried, or mushed) or vegetable (creamed corn on the cob or peaches)

TARGET AREA 5: Visual Logic   Hidden Words

DIRECTIONS: Each line of letters has at least 15 words hidden in it. Look at the letters and write the words as you find them. The letters should stay in the same order and are at least two letters long. See **CLUES** *for help.*

1. **ASHOREASONORTHEME**

_____	_____	_____
_____	_____	_____
_____	_____	_____
_____	_____	_____
_____	_____	_____

2. **PANTHERBITTENSPANKING**

_____	_____	_____
_____	_____	_____
_____	_____	_____
_____	_____	_____
_____	_____	_____

3. **BRACELETTERMINALLOWANCENTER**

4. **TEASEARCHAPLAINCAPABLED**

5. **BADMINTONEWSPAPERMITCH**

6. **ATTACKLEATHERMOMETERRACE**

_____   _____   _____

_____   _____   _____

_____   _____   _____

_____   _____   _____

_____   _____   _____

---

7. **MEDALLIONAMESAKEYELLOW**

_____   _____   _____

_____   _____   _____

_____   _____   _____

_____   _____   _____

---

8. **PAGENTLENDEARMYOURGERMAN**

_____   _____   _____

_____   _____   _____

_____   _____   _____

_____   _____   _____

TARGET AREA 5: Visual Logic

*DIRECTIONS: Each line of letters on the left is hiding a word. If the line of letters is written in the correct grid, a real word will be spelled out in the <u>white</u> boxes. Write the number of the line of letters that fit into that grid to form a word. See **CLUES** for help.*

1. E W E A L R T O Z __

2. S A B T A I N E X __

3. L M P N O I S N T __

4. D E R A N L S E B __

5. S T C O R M I N C __

6. A S K T O I N N G __

7. U W N R D F E H R   ___

8. G R E O L A P E X   ___

9. N E X O R C T A H   ___

10. I D D O E A S T L   ___

11. C H B R A S E I C   ___

12. Q U I L E V R E L   ___

13. F L C R E A S W H   ___

14. A K M R O N I G H   ___

15. E V D I N A Y L P   ___

16. J M O B K E Y R N   ___

17. S L E P A R N E D   ___

18. S C O H A B I G R   ___

19. T H R G I R B L E   ___

20. A G E R C A V E Y   ___

21. L O S T B B E A Y   ___

22. H O U N M B R A N   ___

23. N W E A H R L O Y   ___

24. E S Q B U A S R T   ___

25. A E G W A P K D E   ___

26. T M I C X E A R K   ___

27. L A S T C T O K R ___

28. M O U S S I A C K ___

29. D A J E L M L O Y ___

30. F L I F U T V C H ___

31. Y O R U N G O G Y ___

32. R E E D A S D Y H ___

33. C D H E R I L S D ___

34. P L I O D N G E W ___

35. T F O U R C B H E ___

36. S N E A M R G L Y ___

TARGET AREA 5: Visual Logic   Defined Numbers

DIRECTIONS: *Read the definition and write a number that answers it. See* **CLUES** *for help.*

1. _____   number of toes on one foot

2. _____   number of days in a weekend

3. _____   number of strikes before you are out in baseball

4. _____   number of wheels on a unicycle

5. _____   total number of digits in a phone number

6. _____   number of weeks in a year

7. _____   number of Commandments

8. _____   number of lives a cat is supposed to have

9. _____   number of points on a star

10. _____   number of digits in an original zip code

11. _____   the number 12 in Roman numerals

12. _____   number of ounces in half a pound

13. _____   number of sides on a **STOP** sign

14. _____   number in a trio

15. _____   number of consonants in the word **consonants**

16. _____   number of letters in the alphabet

17. _____ number of cards in a regular deck

18. _____ number of karats in pure gold

19. _____ age you must be in order to vote

20. _____ number of days in February during a leap year

21. _____ number of legs on a dog, a rabbit, and a bird added together

22. _____ number of holes on a regulation golf course

23. _____ number of original colonies in the United States

24. _____ - _____ considered to be perfect vision

25. _____ number of states in America

26. _____ number of days in September, April, June, or November

27. _____ number of days in a year

28. _____ number of dollars in a **grand**

29. _____ number of eyes, fingers, and legs you have added together

30. _____ Farenheit temperature at which water freezes

31. _____ number of things in two dozen

32. _____ number of years in a golden wedding anniversary

33. _____ number of cents in a quarter plus a dime plus a nickel

34. _____ number of letters in your last name

TARGET AREA 5: Visual Logic   Crossword Math

*DIRECTIONS: Solve this puzzle like a regular crossword, except fill in boxes with numbers, not letters. Some of the clues depend on other clues. See **CLUES** for help.*

ACROSS

1. number of days in a year

4. 1 dozen minus 1

6. 400 minus 40

7. 40 minus 1

8. half of 42

11. number of U.S. states

12. number of days in February

14. reverse of **4 down**

15. number between **1 down** and **14 across**

DOWN

1. 30 plus 3

2. 2 times 1 down

3. 1/2 of 1000

4. unlucky number

5. the year of your birth

8. ___ pennies = 1 quarter

9. years in a century plus 3

10. ___ weeks = 1 year

13. **10 down** plus **14 across**

TARGET AREA 5: Visual Logic

Word Searches

*DIRECTIONS: Each page has its own set of directions. On this page, you are given the first letter of the hidden words, the number of letters, and the direction in which they are hidden. Find the word in the grid, circle it, and write the complete word on the lines. See **CLUES** for help.*

ACROSS Left to right

E __ __ __

B __ __ __ __

T __ __ __

R __ __ __

ACROSS Right to left

A __ __ __ __

D __ __ __

K __ __ __ __ __

H __ __ __

DOWN Top to bottom

C __ __ __ __

F __ __

S __ __

M __ __ __

UP Bottom to top

B __ __ __ __ __

F __ __ __

N __ __

U __ __ __

R	E	L	Y	R	E	V
E	Z	O	D	M	I	L
Z	R	U	T	O	S	S
G	G	T	U	O	B	A
E	L	E	N	N	E	K
R	I	A	H	C	P	R
A	M	D	F	A	Q	O
W	B	E	L	T	S	F
E	A	S	Y	C	E	X
B	R	U	K	H	W	B

*The abbreviations (<u>not</u> the words) are hidden in this word search puzzle. Mark the abbreviations as you find them. A second challenge is listed below the first list. See **CLUES** for help.*

S	T	C	Y	K	C	U	T	N	E	K	F
I	M	O	W	B	G	Q	T	W	R	J	O
O	P	S	H	U	X	E	V	A	Y	D	H
N	A	S	J	T	X	N	O	C	A	P	T
I	N	A	D	A	E	T	C	R	M	B	U
L	O	H	S	W	J	S	O	N	G	L	E
L	Z	G	Y	X	I	L	G	K	P	I	S
I	I	O	H	M	O	D	F	S	Y	W	A
X	R	Z	R	C	L	M	J	B	E	F	M
K	A	V	R	B	F	L	O	R	I	D	A

Mark the **abbreviations** in the grid.

association	February	northwest
avenue	highway	package
building	junior	pound
captain	miscellaneous	railroad
etcetera	mountain	Tuesday

Mark the **full name** for the state in the grid.

AZ	FL	IL	NY
CO	GA	KY	TX

Workbook for Cognitive Skills copyright © Susan Howell Brubaker 2009

This word search puzzle is a little different. The words are made up of arrows plus words. For example, the phrase "right-of-way" would look like "→OFWAY" in the grid. The top of each column shows the symbol that is part of each word below it. The words can be hidden in any direction. Mark each word as you find it. See CLUES for help.

T	O	U	C	H	↓	B	→	↑	F	B	V	M	Q
P	L	→	X	A	E	N	R	U	T	←	A	U	E
↑	A	↓	R	→	I	P	V	S	D	K	→	C	↑
Y	C	←	P	A	L	A	T	E	E	O	H	N	Q
X	↑	I	C	O	↑	I	B	↑	Y	F	I	W	H
D	C	T	V	F	U	Z	↓	N	S	Y	X	O	T
E	A	S	←	I	N	R	B	G	↑	I	←	T	E
D	K	R	N	E	L	P	←	U	E	↓	D	↓	S
N	E	M	→	E	↓	→	Y	S	C	M	O	E	↑
A	G	F	A	T	D	O	S	R	←	K	A	I	↓
H	F	↑	N	Y	←	F	I	E	L	D	L	T	S
←	L	U	G	Q	J	W	↓	V	I	↓	L	E	R
N	O	↓	L	O	T	A	M	O	P	B	→	Q	↑
C	U	M	E	↓	W	Y	H	←	Z	↑	K	P	H

→ = right	← = left	↑ = up	↓ = down

all right	cleft palate	buckle up	countdown
civil rights	left field	cupcake	downpour
frighten	left-handed	makeup	downtown
right angle	leftovers	upset	lie down
right-of-way	left turn	upside down	touchdown

Workbook for Cognitive Skills copyright © Susan Howell Brubaker 2009

TARGET AREA 5: Visual Logic

DIRECTIONS: *Enter the words from the bottom of the pages into the grid to form a crossword reading across and down. A few letters have been inserted to get you started. See* **CLUES** *for help.*

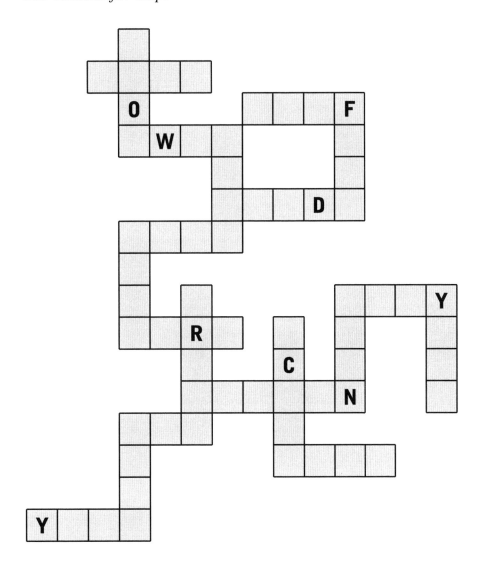

crust	leaf	roar	star
earn	note	scare	trade
easy	open	set	twin
edit	rare	spot	yarn
fire	rate	sprain	your

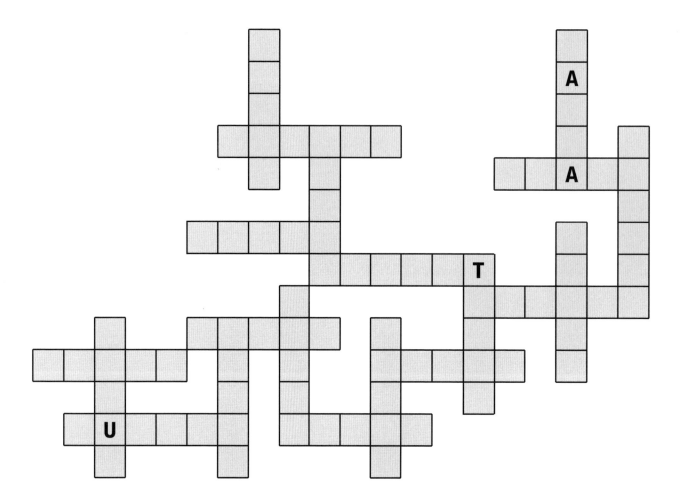

apple	guava	limes	roast
bread	honey	muffin	salad
candy	icing	nachos	toast
decaf	jelly	orange	waffle
flour	kiwis	pasta	yogurt

TARGET AREA 6:
Logical Solutions

TARGET AREA 6: Logical Solutions   Context Clues

*DIRECTIONS: Each question gives five clues that describe a common item. The box represents the name of the item. Write its name as soon as you know what it is. See **CLUES** for help.*

1. ☐ would be stored in the kitchen.

   Most children do not like the taste of ☐ unless it is sweetened.

   The sale of ☐ is a multi-billion dollar industry.

   ☐ is a popular flavor for beverages, candy and ice cream.

   It seems like every town has at least one ☐ shop.

   What is the word? _____

2. Usually people keep a supply of ☐ at home.

   You can buy ☐ in different colors, sizes, and shapes.

   ☐ are made from paper or plastic.

   When you buy greeting cards, ☐ are usually included.

   If an ☐ doesn't have adhesive, you might lick it to seal it.

   What is the word? _____

3. ☐ comes in different sizes and shapes.

   ☐s are used for decoration as well as for function.

   Most cars have at least three ☐ in or on them.

   Everyone should look in a ☐ at least once a day.

   Large ☐ can be hung on the wall and small ones fit easily in your hand.

   What is the word? _____

---

4. Most ☐ are kept in a closet.

   ☐ are made from materials such as leather, fur, or foam.

   Children will outgrow their ☐, but adults normally do not.

   ☐ are usually not made to be worn outdoors.

   Although ☐ were meant to be worn morning and night, many people wear them any time.

   What is the word? _____

---

5. Most people love ☐.

   Many foods are flavored or covered with some form of ☐.

   ☐ can be in solid, liquid, or powdered form.

   Small pieces of ☐ can be mixed into ice cream or cookies.

   ☐ is used in making truffles, mousse, and tortes.

   What is the word? _____

6. Everybody has a ☐ and each person's is a little different.

You use your ☐ every day of your life.

Researchers love to study the ☐.

The ☐ controls your thoughts and actions.

Your skull protects your ☐ from being hurt or damaged.

What is the word? _____

---

7. ☐ are popular hostess gifts.

In colonial times, ☐ were needed household items.

Crafty people make ☐ to use, give away, or sell.

Romantic dinners often include ☐ on the table.

Some ☐ give off a pleasant scent when they are lit.

What is the word? _____

---

8. We all ☐ at one time or another.

Sometimes a ☐ accompanies a cold.

A ☐ starts with an irritation in your throat.

Smoking often causes a distinctive ☐.

Losenges or ☐ syrup may help a ☐.

What is the word? _____

9. Originally ☐ were made for prospectors in the 1800s.

   Today ☐ are made for everyone of all ages.

   The most popular ☐ color continues to be blue.

   ☐ are made from other materials in addition to denim.

   Although ☐ can fade, they never seem to fade from fashion.

   What is the word? _____

---

10. ☐ grows in many climates around the world.

    ☐ needs water to keep it from turning brown.

    Fertilizer helps prevent weeds from growing in ☐.

    ☐ can be grown from seed or sod.

    It is popular for ☐ to be kept cut around a home.

    What is the word? _____

---

11. ☐s are worn by some animals as well as people.

    A bone in your body has ☐ in its name.

    A priest's ☐ looks different from one you might wear.

    A shirt or blouse can have a ☐.

    A leash attaches to a dog's ☐.

    What is the word? _____

TARGET AREA 6: Logical Solutions Letter Words

DIRECTIONS: *The letters and numbers represent words that <u>sound</u> like that letter or number when it is heard. Hyphenated letters or numbers are pronounced together to make one word and double letters are pronounced as if they were plural (BB=bees). Write the sentence that is represented by what you hear when the letters and numbers are said aloud. See* **CLUES** *for help.*

1. I O U 4 D PP.

_____

2. I C Y U 1 N M-E.

_____

3. J S D 1 2 X-QQ.

_____

4. I M 2 D-Z 2 C.

_____

5. I C A B N D I-V.

_____

6. R U 2 B-Z 2 C D 10-R?

_____

7. L-X 00 K-C 4 D D-J.

_____

8. U R 8-T N U R YY.

_____

9. RR S D 1 2 B B-10.

_____

10. CC D S-K-P B-4 N-E-1 CC.

_____

11. I M A 4-N-R 2 U.

_____

12. I 8 B-4 N-E-1.

_____

13. 10-S S E-Z 4 U.

_____

TARGET AREA 6: Logical Solutions   Homonym Sentences

DIRECTIONS: Homonyms are words that sound the same but are spelled differently. If you said each sentence aloud, it would sound like a normal sentence. Write the sentence that is represented but use the homonym spelling so it makes sense. The few underlined words should not be changed. See CLUES for help.

1. Aisle bye flours four yore ant.

   _____

2. Fore sail: gnu quarts wring. Cheep.

   _____

3. Hour sun flue too Bolder Damn Sundae.

   _____

4. Eye oh ewe four Peat's gnu blew genes.

   _____

5. Due knot waist watt ewe urn.

   _____

6. The night maid eh soared four the prints.

   _____

7. Eye new wee wood knot bee aloud two serf.

   _____

8. Ant Genie maid chilly four Kneel.

   _____

9. Eye tolled ewe knot two lye too hymn.

_____

10. Wee tract to bares scene inn <u>the</u> woulds.

_____

11. There crews sales passed Roam <u>and</u> Grease.

_____

12. Hues ant mussed finnish rapping <u>the</u> pries.

_____

13. Eye herd roomers Rustle ode sum cache.

_____

14. Pleas chews witch flower too yews inn yore bred.

_____

15. Eye guest <u>my</u> suite ant inn Main died <u>her</u> hare.

_____

16. Pleas titan yore hoarses rains.

_____

17. Witch won wood bee <u>the</u> mustered too bye?

_____

DIRECTIONS: *Each question gives a different and unusual definition for one of the words in the box. Write the word on the line as you use it. Each word is used once. See* **CLUES** *for help.*

AJAR	**LEGEND**
MINIMUM	**HIJACK**
CAPSIZE	**CARROT**
FORBID	**TENANTS**

1. A greeting to a friend _____

2. A very small flower _____

3. One more than nine ants _____

4. What you need to know in order to buy a hat _____

5. An item similar to a bottle _____

6. Your foot begins at this point _____

7. Rust does this to your automobile _____

8. Items in an auction are this _____

NOVICES	REBELLION	CONFINED
PUPPET	ISLAND	THINKING
BARRACKS	KIDNAP	EVEREST
HERRING	REARRANGE	MISTRUST

1. a nonconformist king of beasts _____

2. what Adam's wife did after working in the garden _____

3. the stove in back of the others _____

4. corrosion in a very humid climate _____

5. a piece of woman's jewelry _____

6. what a child takes in the afternoon _____

7. where wine glasses are stored _____

8. it is not water; it _____

9. this describes the perfect person _____

10. prisoner who had to pay for breaking the rules _____

11. stuffed animal that a dog plays with _____

12. ruler who could gain a few pounds _____

TARGET AREA 6: Logical Solutions   Word Similarities

DIRECTIONS: The words on each line have something in common. Decide how they appear to be alike and write it on the line. The meanings of the words are not important to the answers. See **CLUES** *for help.*

1. dribble   butter   collar   book   drummer

2. defeat   study   hijack   nope   stubborn

3. dread   high   species   treat   window

4. bubble   nodded   pepper   fluffy   throttle

5. gypsy   myth   spry   cyst   rhythm

6. oh   pea   bee   eye   cue

7. banana   criticism   delete   untruthful   cocoon

_____

8. setter   street   trees   steer   tresses

_____

9. allspice   popcorn   freshman   bobcat   windshield

_____

10. pat   bill   jack   sue   ray

_____

11. sew   though   know   doe   go

_____

12. lull   noon   Anna   sass   deed

_____

13. gag   refer   level   did   sexes

_____

14. I   in   gin   grin   grind

_____

TARGET AREA 6: Logical Solutions   Calendar Dates

*DIRECTIONS: Use the calendar below to answer the questions. Your answer will be a date on the calendar. See **CLUES** for help.*

SUN.	MON.	TUES.	WED.	THURS.	FRI.	SAT.
		1	2	3	4	5
6	7	8	9	10	11	12
13	14	15	16	17	18	19
20	21	22	23	24	25	26
27	28	29	30	31		

1. The date is not during the first or last week of the month.

    It is during the weekend.

    It is before the 20th.

    It is not during the second weekend of the month.

    It is not on a Sunday.

    What is the date being described? _____

2. The date is not on a weekend.

   It is not during the second week of the month.

   It is between the 21st and the 25th.

   It is in the middle of the week.

   It is an odd, not even, numbered date.

   What is the date being described? _____

---

3. The date is on a Monday.

   It is not the 28th.

   It is not in the third week of the month.

   It is a single digit number.

   What is the date being described? _____

---

4. The date is a number that can be divided by two.

   It is a day during the week, not on the weekend.

   It is during the last week of the month.

   Four months have this number of days in them; all the other months
   have more or fewer days in them.

   What is the date being described? _____

5. The date is not in the first or the last week of the month.

   It is not on a Thursday.

   It is not a number in the twenties.

   It is an even number.

   It is not a one-digit number.

   It is not the 13th, the 16th, or the 18th.

   It is not the day following any of those three days.

   It is not on a Friday.

   What is the date being described? _____

---

6. The date is in the first half of the month.

   It is not on a day beginning with the letter T.

   It is not in the middle of the week.

   It is between the answer to number 1 and the answer to number 5.

   It is an odd-numbered day.

   What is the date being described? _____

TARGET AREA 6: Logical Solutions Letter Tracking

DIRECTIONS: In each group, form words reading down by following the directions and using the grid. See **CLUES** for help.

O	F	C	R
G	Y	N	A
L	P	D	U

1. Start with **C** ____

   Go left 2 ____

   Go down 2 and right 1 ____

   Go up 1 ____

2. Start with **Y** ____

   Go right 2 ____

   Go up 1 ____

   Go left 1 and down 2 ____

3. <u>Start with **A**</u>   _____

    Go down 1 and left 3   _____

    Go up 2   _____

    Go right 2 and down 1   _____

    Go left 2   _____

---

4. <u>Start with **F**</u>   _____

    Go right 2   _____

    Go down 2   _____

    Go left 3 and up 1   _____

    Go right 3   _____

    Go down 1 and left 3   _____

---

5. <u>Start with **D**</u>   _____

    Go up 2 and right 1   _____

    Go down 1   _____

    Go left 3   _____

    Go up 1   _____

    Go right 2 and down 1   _____

TARGET AREA 6: Logical Solutions   Directional Words

DIRECTIONS: In each group, form words reading down by following the directions and using the grid. See CLUES for help.

O	E	A	L
B	T	I	G
D	N	H	R

1. Start with **B**   ____

    Go north 1 and east 2   ____

    Go south 2 and east 1   ____

    Go west 2   ____

---

2. Start with **H**   ____

    Go north 2 and west 1   ____

    Go west 1 and south 2   ____

    Go east 3 and north 1   ____

    Go north 1 and west 2   ____

3. <u>Start with **N**</u> _____

    Go west 1 and north 2 _____

    Go south 1 and east 1 _____

    Go east 1 _____

    Go south 1 and west 1 _____

    Go east 2 and north 1 _____

---

4. <u>Start with **G**</u> _____

    Go south 1 _____

    Go west 1 and north 1 _____

    Go west 1 and south 1 _____

    Go west 1 _____

---

5. <u>Start with **D**</u> _____

    Go north 2 and east 2 _____

    Go south 2 and west 1 _____

    Go east 2 and north 1 _____

    Go west 2 and north 1 _____

    Go east 2 and south 2 _____

TARGET AREA 6: Logical Solutions   Letters by Location

*DIRECTIONS: In each group, form words reading down by following the directions and using the grid. See **CLUES** for help.*

P	H	M	C
D	A	S	B
V	R	L	E

1. The first letter is between **H** and **R**.   ____

    The second letter is in the top right corner.   ____

    The third letter is directly below **A**.   ____

    The fourth letter is in the bottom right corner.   ____

---

2. The first letter is above and to the right of **D**.   ____

    The second letter is below and to the right of **S**.   ____

    The third letter is below and to the left of **B**.   ____

    The fourth letter is above and to the left of **A**.   ____

3. The first letter is in the lower left corner. _____

   The second letter is in the lower right corner. _____

   The third letter is between **L** and **V**. _____

   The fourth letter is between **C** and **E**. _____

---

4. The first letter is below **P** and above **V**. _____

   The second letter is to the left of **L**. _____

   The third letter is below **B**. _____

   The fourth letter is below **H** and above **R**. _____

   The fifth letter is between **H** and **C**. _____

---

5. The first letter is surrounded by **B**, **A**, **L**, **M**. _____

   The second letter is surrounded by **B**, **L**, **S**. _____

   The third letter is surrounded by **H**, **D**, **S**, **R**. _____

   The fourth letter is surrounded by **V**, **A**, **L**. _____

   The fifth letter is surrounded by **M**, **S**, **B**. _____

   The sixth letter is surrounded by **P**, **A**, **M**. _____

Refer to the grid to answer the questions. A row goes across, and a column goes down. <u>*A line*</u> <u>*refers to either a row or a column.*</u>

W	I	A	J	E	S
R	M	C	H	L	P
D	S	T	B	E	V
F	P	Y	R	G	O
R	R	N	T	K	U
E	D	A	G	I	C

1. What are the only two side-by-side vowels? _____

2. Which line contains just the first half of the alphabet? _____

3. Which line contains only letters that look the same as capital or lowercase letters? _____

4. What are the third and fourth letters in the line that begins and ends with the same letter? _____

5. Which letter is repeated the most? _____

6. Which lines have no vowels? _____

Use the grid on page 286 to find the letters. The answers will form a word reading down.

7. First letter: fourth column, first letter   _____

   Second letter: fourth row, last letter   _____

   Third letter: third column, fourth letter   _____

   Fourth letter: fourth row, first letter   _____

   Fifth letter: last column, second to last letter   _____

   Sixth letter: second row, fifth letter   _____

---

8. The first letter is between **C** and **L**.   _____

   The second letter is a vowel and has a vowel below it.   _____

   The third letter is above **A**.   _____

   The fourth letter is in a corner.   _____

   The fifth letter is above a **P** in two places.   _____

   The last letter is in both the third and fourth columns.   _____

TARGET AREA 6: Logical Solutions   Sudoku

DIRECTIONS: Each large box is made up of six smaller boxes. Each of these smaller boxes and each row going across and each column going down must contain the letters or numbers as indicated. Each number or letter can only appear once within the six boxes, only once in each row and once in each column. Fill in the missing letters or numbers. See CLUES for help.

Fill in the numbers from **1** to **6**.

2		3	4	1	
5	1		3		2
		6	5	2	1
1	5	2			3
	2	5		3	4
3	4		2	5	6

Fill in the numbers from **57** to **62**.

	59	58	62	57	60
57	62		59		58
62	58	61	60	59	
59		57	58		61
58	61		57	60	
60		59		58	

Continue, but fill in the missing letters (alphabetical order).

Fill in the numbers from **A** to **I**.

F	D		C	E	
C	E	A	D		B
E	C	F		A	
	B		E	C	F
D	A	E		B	C
B		C	A		E

Fill in the letters from **K** to **P**.

M	P		N		K
	K	O	L	M	
L	O	N		P	
P			O	N	L
K	N	M		L	O
		P	M	K	N

TARGET AREA 6: Logical Solutions   Map Routes

DIRECTIONS: Answer the questions by using the information on the map. Several routes are possible. Choose the most direct route. See **CLUES** *for help.*

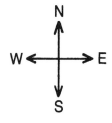

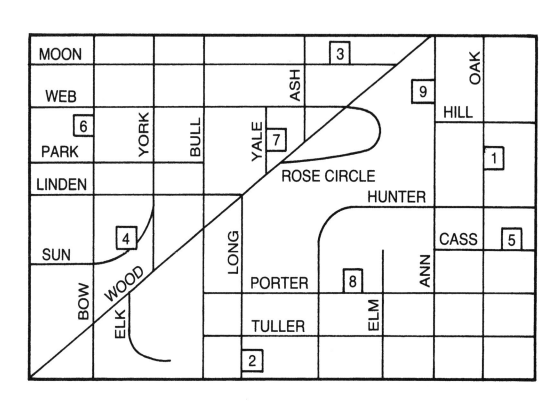

1. Write out how you would go from number **1** to **2**.

_____

_____

2. go from number **2** to **3**

_____

_____

3. Write out how you would go from number **7** to **2**.

_____

_____

4. go from number **5** to **6**

_____

_____

5. go from number **6** to **9**

_____

_____

6. go from number **3** to **8**

_____

_____

7. go from number **4** to **5**

_____

_____

8. go from number **1** to **6**

_____

_____

TARGET AREA 6: Logical Solutions

Map Reading

*DIRECTIONS: Use the map to answer the questions. See **CLUES** for help.*

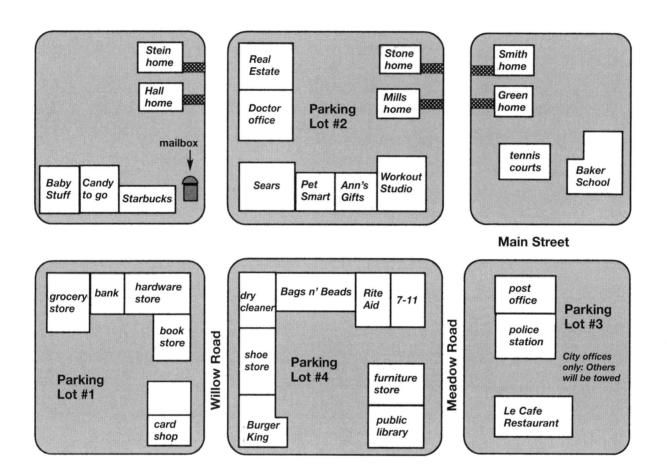

1. If you were going to the shoe store, which parking lot would you use?

_____

2. The hardware store is at the intersection of what two streets?

_____

3. What is between the place where you could buy a hamster and the place where you could lift weights?

_____

4. Who lives closer to the bank—the Steins or the Stones?

_____

5. Mr. Green wants to walk to Sears. What route should he take?

_____

6. Exactly where is the vacant store located?

_____

7. Name all the places you could buy coffee and a muffin.

_____

8. Where might you be going if you parked in Lot #3?

_____

9. If a group wanted to leave school and get some candy, how many streets would they have to cross to get there?

_____

10. If you were at the drugstore, would it be closer for you to mail a letter at the mailbox or at the post office?

   _____

11. If you were leaving Ann's Gifts, what would be the closest place to buy a newspaper?

   _____

12. Neither Lisa Hall nor Joan Mills is allowed to cross the street by herself. Which girl can go to the candy store alone?

   _____

13. What is the exact location of the bank?

   _____

14. You are in Lot #2. In what order would you go to the following places before returning to your car?

   _____ Candy to go   _____ Card shop

   _____ Furniture store   _____ Baby Stuff

15. What is between where you could get your sweater cleaned and where you could buy a Whopper?

   _____

TARGET AREA 6: Logical Solutions   Map Construction

DIRECTIONS: *Determine the name of each street on the map and write it on the line next to its*
*number. Use the clues on the next page to figure out the street names. The **first***
*time a street is named, it is underlined. See **CLUES** for help.*

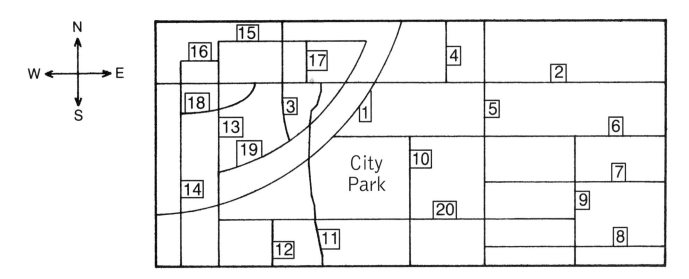

1. _____

2. _____

3. _____

4. _____

5. _____

6. _____

7. _____

8. _____

9. _____

10. _____

11. _____

12. _____

13. _____

14. _____

15. _____

16. _____

17. _____

18. _____

19. _____

20. _____

1. <u>Cranbrook</u> is street number 2.

2. <u>Sunset</u> is the only street that begins at Cranbrook and winds its way south to the end of the map.

3. <u>Redding</u> starts at Cranbrook and goes to the north border of the map.

4. The road farthest to the west running north and south is **Verona**.

5. <u>Newgate</u> is street number 13.

6. <u>Drake</u> begins at Verona and ends at Cranbrook.

7. <u>Fairview</u> is east of Redding and crosses Cranbrook going from the north to the southern border of the map.

8. Both <u>Walnut</u> and <u>Hillside</u> begin at Fairview and run east to the end of the map. Walnut is two blocks north of Hillside.

9. <u>Kinross</u> is a short street connecting Newgate and Verona.

10. <u>Springer</u> forms the eastern border of the City Park.

11. <u>Troy</u> is a curved street running between the west and north ends of the map.

12. <u>Birwood</u> runs east and west between Newgate and **Oxford**.

13. Sunset crosses Oxford, <u>Troy</u>, and <u>Woodlawn</u> as it moves south.

14. Woodlawn forms the southern boundary of the City Park and runs between Newgate and <u>Pine</u>.

15. <u>Greenfield</u> is bounded by Birwood and Cranbrook.

16. <u>Lakeland</u>, <u>Lincoln</u>, and <u>Maple</u> are the remaining streets not yet named.

17. Maple is the only street of these three that runs east and west.

18. Lakeland ends at Oxford.

TARGET AREA 6: Logical Solutions

Map Locations

DIRECTIONS: Use the map below to answer the questions. Write the number of the location that fits the description. See **CLUES** for help.

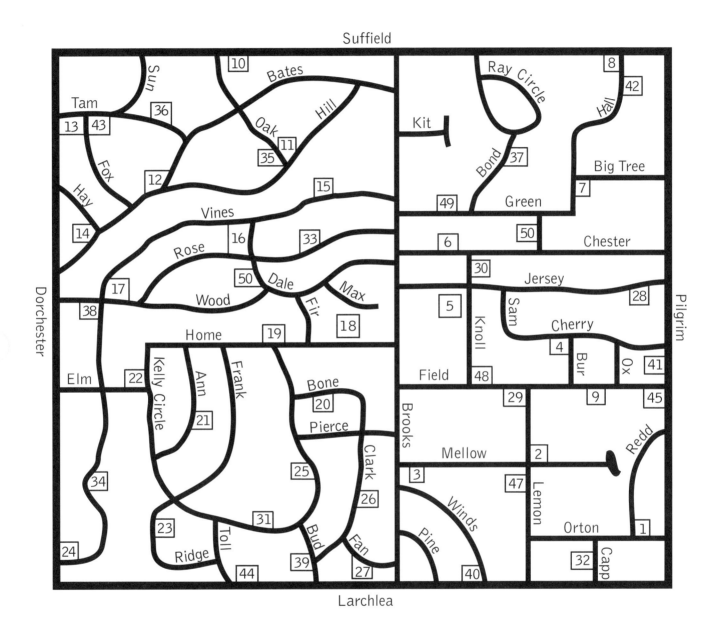

1. It is at the intersection of Hay and Hill. _____

2. It is bounded by Field, Cherry, and Pilgrim. _____

3. It is between Bur and Ox. _____

Workbook for Cognitive Skills copyright © Susan Howell Brubaker 2009

4. It is on the street between Kelly Circle and Frank. _____

5. It is the most northern spot west of Brooks. _____

6. It is on a short street that does not have a name. _____

7. It is the only location on Clark. _____

8. It is on Tam closest to Bates. _____

9. It is south of Jersey, north of Field, and west of Knoll. _____

10. It is on the south side of Wood. _____

11. It is at Bates and Hill. _____

12. It is between Fir and Frank. _____

13. It is south of Orton and east of Winds. _____

14. It is on Hall but not on a corner. _____

15. Clark dead ends at this point. _____

16. It is north of Bud and south of Pierce on Kelly. _____

17. It is where streets beginning with **O** and **R** meet. _____

TARGET AREA 6: Logical Solutions

Codes

DIRECTIONS: *There are different codes in each exercise. Use the information to figure out the code, then write one letter per line. Your answers will make a message.* See **CLUES** *for help.*

CODE 1: Each number stands for a letter in the alphabet starting in order from 1 to 26.

A	B	C	D	E	F	G	H	I	J	K	L	M

N	O	P	Q	R	S	T	U	V	W	X	Y	Z

M Y   D O C T O R   P U T   M E
13 25   4 15 3 20 15 18   16 21 20   13 5

O N   A   S E A F O O D
15 14   1   19 5 1 6 15 15 4

D I E T.   N O W   I   O N L Y
4 9 5 20   14 15 23   9   15 14 12 25

E A T   W H E N   I   S E E
5 1 20   23 8 5 14   9   19 5 5

F O O D.
6 15 15 4

CODE 2: Transfer the first letter of each word in the paragraph to the lines in order to form a message.

Turnovers, hamburgers, enchiladas, mousse, and I like indulging. Some students of suppers linger over what to have and taste. They have every food looked over well. Each restaurant should end evening dinners successfully. In offering recipes, diners each receive exciting descriptions and rare reproductions. I view each dinner as stimulating. A banquet of unusual quality uncovers enormous treasures.

___ ___ ___ ___   ___ ___ ___ ___ ___   ___ ___ ___   ___ ___ ___

___ ___ ___ ___ ___   ___ ___ ___ ___   ___ ___ ___ ___

___ ___ ___ ___ ___   ___ ___ ___ ___ ___   ___

___ ___ ___ ___ ___ ___ ___   ___ ___ ___ ___ ___ ___

___ ___   ___   ___ ___ ___ ___ ___ ___ ___ .

CODE 3: Transfer the last letter of each word in the paragraph to the lines in order to form a message.

Hold me. If I can, I rest. I do clean—no half a job. Go over where it's too warm. We do frown. We draw with no brush. Area bankers can go without cash. I can bring it also. It's a crazy job. You can't cross a busy boss. I met a man, many saw a boy.

___ ___ ___ ___ ___ ___ ___ ___ ___ ___   ___ ___   ___

___ ___ ___ ___ :   ___ ___ ___ ___ ___ ___ ___   ___ ___ ___

___ ___ ___   ___ ___ ___ ___ ___   ___ ___

___ ___ ___ ___   ___ ___ ___   ___ ___ ___

___ ___ ___ ___ ___ ___ .

TARGET AREA 6: Logical Solutions   Project Planning

*DIRECTIONS: Each page presents a different dilemma. The instructions appear below each diagram. The <u>**first**</u> time an item to be placed in the diagram is mentioned, it is **bolded** and <u>underlined</u>. Fill in the diagram so everything fits the facts. See **CLUES** for help.*

JAN'S CLOSET

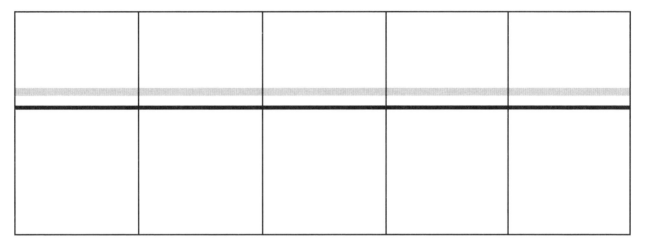

Jan needs to organize her closet so she can find things better. Five things will go on the shelves (gray line) above the area where the clothes will hang (black line). Write the names of the articles in the boxes where they belong.

1. Jan wants her **<u>blouses</u>** to be the first things hanging on the left and her **<u>jackets</u>** to be the last things hanging on the right.

2. **<u>Scarves</u>** will be in boxes in the middle of the closet.

3. **<u>Slacks</u>** will be hung next to her jackets and directly below her **<u>belts</u>**.

4. **<u>Gloves</u>** will be on the shelf between her **<u>socks</u>** and scarves.

5. **<u>Skirts</u>** will go below the gloves and to the left of the **<u>dresses</u>**.

6. Jan's **<u>hats</u>** will go in the only remaining space on the shelf.

KITCHEN SHELVES

TOP

MIDDLE

BOTTOM

The kitchen shelves are divided into 12 areas as shown above. Each area will hold some type of food. Put the underlined foods in their proper places according to the information given.

1. I use **vegetables** a lot, so they should be on a bottom shelf.

2. I want the **snacks** to be on a top shelf so I won't be tempted by them.

3. The **cat food** should be on the bottom shelf on the left end, and the **spices** directly above it.

4. The top shelf on the right should hold **cookies**, with **crackers** to the left of them on the shelf below.

5. **Cake mixes** belong above the crackers and the **coffee** below them.

6. Canned **fruit** goes between the spices and crackers.

7. Snacks go directly above the fruit.

8. The vegetables should be just below the **cereal**, which is on the second shelf.

9. **Pasta** should be kept on a higher shelf than the **soup**.

COURTYARD MALL

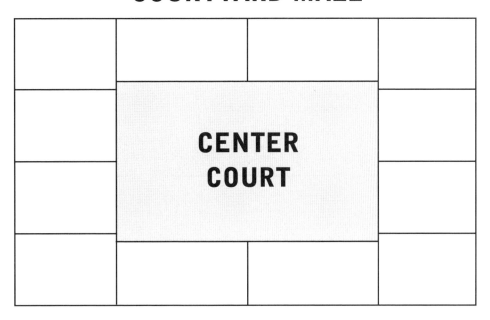

Below is a list of the stores that are planning to move into Courtyard Mall. Using the information, decide where each store should go, and write the name of the store in the correct box. There is more than one possible arrangement.

Arby's—food
Better Vision—eye care
Breyer's—ice cream
Burt's—books
Dexter's—shoes
Dimensions—clothing

Flora's—flowers
Gap—clothing
Hallmark—cards
Kidland—toys
Macy's—department store
Penney's—department store

1. The clothing stores should be diagonally across the court from each other and so should the department stores.

2. **Hallmark** should be next to a restaurant.

3. **Arby's** will do well if it is next to the **Gap**.

4. The bookstore and the florist should be between **Penney's** and **Dimensions**.

5. **Kidland** should be directly across the Center Court from Arby's.

6. **Dexter's** should not be next to a toy store or any place that sells food.

GARDEN PLOT

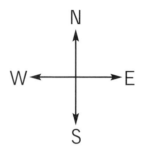

Each box in the diagram represents a plot for a specific vegetable to be grown. Based on the information below, fill in each box with the name of a vegetable.

1. The **tomatoes** on stakes should go in the most northeastern plot so that they will not shade the rest of the vegetables.

2. The **cucumbers** and **squash** will spread out so each should be on a corner spot on the south side of the garden.

3. The **lettuce** should go between the cucumbers and squash because the lettuce will be harvested early so the cucumbers and squash will have room to spread out.

4. The **pumpkins** will take up two plots along the north end of the garden.

5. The two center spots that do not border on the outside should be **broccoli** and **cauliflower**, with the broccoli just south of the pumpkins.

6. Plant the **onions** north of the squash and next to the cauliflower.

7. The **green peppers** will grow well between the tomatoes and onions.

8. The **peas** should be planted to the south of the **beans** where they will get more sun.

FAMILY TREE

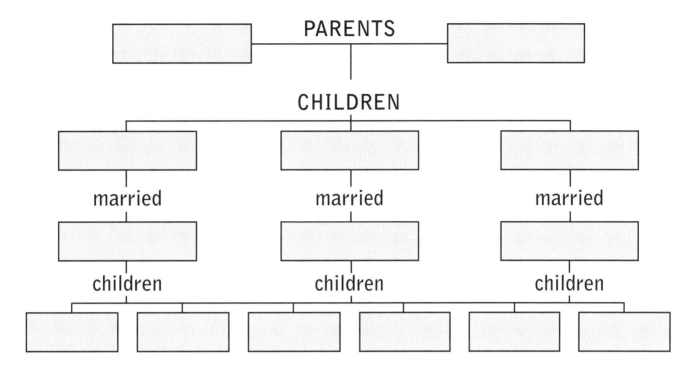

The chart shows that Christopher and Barbara had three children. Each child married and had two children. Using the information below, put the names in their correct boxes.

The parents had one girl named **Linda** and two boys.

Jeff has a boy and a girl whose names start with the same letter.

Kevin's uncles are **Ed** and **Robert**.

Brian and **Jason** are brothers.

Linda and Ed's daughter's name ends in a vowel.

Carrie married someone whose name has the same number of letters as hers.

Only one family has children who are of the same sex.

Mary's daughter is **Katy**.

Alex and **Lori** are twins.

TARGET AREA 6: Logical Solutions   Schedule Planning

DIRECTIONS: *Each page presents a different situation. The instructions are given below the diagram. The **first** time an item to be scheduled is listed, it is **bolded** and* <u>underlined</u>*. Fill in the diagram so everything fits the facts. See **CLUES** for help.*

MARY'S SCHEDULE

9:00 _____

9:30 _____

10:00 _____

10:30 _____

11:00 _____

11:30 _____

12:00 _____

Mary wants to plan her morning so she can finish her errands by noon, when she is to meet a friend for **lunch**. She needs to take her sweaters and drop them off at the **dry cleaners**. The **shoe repair shop** and **bank** don't open until 10:00. The **post office** and **bakery** are closest to Mary's home, and they are also open the earliest. There is usually a line at the post office by 9:30, so Mary likes to get there before then. Mary wants to be at the bank when it opens. The shoe repair shop is next to the restaurant where she is having lunch. Mary plans on being at the **library** at 11:00.

TOUR OF NEW YORK CITY

Stop 1 _____

Stop 2 _____

Stop 3 _____

Stop 4 _____

Stop 5 _____

Stop 6 _____

Stop 7 _____

Bob's sister is coming to visit him in New York City. He wants to give her a day's tour of the city. Bob thought his sister should see the **Museum of Art** and **Rockefeller Center** in the morning. They want to shop on **5th Avenue** right after they see **Times Square**. They are having **lunch** at a restaurant near **Central Park**, so they can walk off their meal in the park. Bob plans to take his sister to the top of the **Empire State Building** first, so he can point out the places they will visit later in the day. After seeing the Museum of Art, they will have lunch. They will walk through Central Park before hailing a cab to Times Square.

TALENT SHOW ACTS

Act 1 _____

Act 2 _____

Act 3 _____

Act 4 _____

Act 5 _____

Act 6 _____

Act 7 _____

Act 8 _____

The producer of the Noville's Talent Show has seven acts and an **intermission** to schedule. The **magician** and the **ventriloquist** must go on before the intermission because they have another show to do later that night. The piano for the **pianist** will be brought on stage during the intermission. The **Scottish Dancers** volunteered to be the first act. There are three acts scheduled after the intermission. The **Barbershop Quartet** will perform during the first part of the show. They sing after the ventriloquist and before the magician. The piano has to be removed from the stage before the **juggler** can perform. The **comedian** will follow the pianist.

SCHEDULE FOR FURNITURE DELIVERY

Stop 1 _____

Stop 2 _____

Stop 3 _____

Stop 4 _____

Stop 5 _____

Stop 6 _____

Stop 7 _____

Stop 8 _____

The Stuft Furniture Store needs to plan its deliveries a day ahead. All deliveries are scheduled so that the least amount of time is wasted. The items that are packed on the truck first are scheduled to be delivered last, while the things packed last will be delivered first. Last Saturday the schedule went as follows:

The **dining room table** was delivered immediately after the **couch**. The **recliner** was the first stop. The **wall unit** was the fifth stop of the day. The **bedroom suite** was packed on the truck first. The **desk** was loaded just in front of it. The **loveseat** was delivered on the stop before the couch. **Bookcases** were also delivered that day.

TARGET AREA 6: Logical Solutions   Logic Problems

DIRECTIONS: *Each chart will help you figure out the answer based on information from the clues. As you read a clue, decide if a fact belongs with a person. If it does, circle that word on the person's line and cross it out as a choice on the other lines. If you know a fact does not belong with a person, cross it out on that person's line. Your answers must fit all the facts. See* **CLUES** *for help.*

OWNER	TYPE OF DOG			
Amy	beagle	cocker	dachshund	Gt. Dane
Joe	beagle	cocker	dachshund	Gt. Dane
John	beagle	cocker	dachshund	Gt. Dane
Mary	beagle	cocker	dachshund	Gt. Dane

Determine the type of dog each person owns.

1. A man has the largest dog, and a woman has the dog with the shortest legs.

2. Mary does not own the cocker.

3. John's beagle, Mitzi, likes to play with Dandy, Mary's dog.

4. Amy's type of dog has six letters in it.

NAME	JOB			
Barb	artist	banker	manager	writer
Bob	artist	banker	manager	writer
Sam	artist	banker	manager	writer
Sue	artist	banker	manager	writer

Determine what job each person does.

1. The artist and the banker often meet Sue for lunch.

2. The manager is not a woman, and the banker is not a man.

3. Sam works in his basement studio.

NAME	AGE			
Chris	25	30	40	50
Dave	25	30	40	50
Lori	25	30	40	50
Pat	25	30	40	50

Determine how old each person is.

1. Lori is half as old as Chris.

2. Dave is older than Pat, but he is not as old as Chris.

NAME	VACATION SPOT			
Baker	Chicago	L.A.	NYC	Toronto
Davis	Chicago	L.A.	NYC	Toronto
Smith	Chicago	L.A.	NYC	Toronto
Turner	Chicago	L.A.	NYC	Toronto

All of the couples live in Florida and are planning a trip somewhere they have never been. Determine who is going where.

1. The Bakers are looking forward to seeing the leaves change color.

2. The Smiths have been to both Toronto and Chicago on previous trips.

3. The Turners hope to have time to spend a day at Disneyland.

4. The Davis family will need passports for their trip.

NAME	DINNER			
Megan	fish	pizza	ham	steak
Greg	fish	pizza	ham	steak
Kate	fish	pizza	ham	steak
Nick	fish	pizza	ham	steak

Determine what each person had for dinner. They all chose different meals, and all enjoyed their choices very much.

1. Megan does not like ham.

2. Nick does not like steak or ham.

3. Kate had salmon for dinner.

WIFE	HUSBAND			
Anna	Andy	Mike	Sam	Tom
Jenny	Andy	Mike	Sam	Tom
Emily	Andy	Mike	Sam	Tom
Sarah	Andy	Mike	Sam	Tom

Determine the names of the couples.

1. Andy and Emily live next door to each other.
2. Mike and his wife have one child and Jenny and her husband have two girls.
3. Sarah and her husband have a dog, but no children.
4. Neither Tom nor Andy have a pet.
5. Jenny and Andy play poker with Mike and his wife twice a month.
6. Tom is not married to Emily.

OWNER	HOUSE COLOR			
Howe	blue	green	tan	white
Jones	blue	green	tan	white
Pratt	blue	green	tan	white
Walker	blue	green	tan	white

Determine the color of each family's house.

1. The Pratts live in a green two-story colonial.
2. The Jones' house is not tan.
3. The white house was just built last year.
4. The blue house does not belong to the Howes.
5. The Walker and the Howe houses are 30 years old.

NAME	CITY			
Bud	San Diego	St. Louis	Atlanta	Miami
Joe	San Diego	St. Louis	Atlanta	Miami
Al	San Diego	St. Louis	Atlanta	Miami
Ed	San Diego	St. Louis	Atlanta	Miami

Determine where each man lives.

1. Ed does not live on the east or west coast.

2. Joe lives the closest to Las Vegas.

3. In one case, the name and the city start with the same letter.

FIRST	LAST NAME			
Jean	Clark	Johnson	Marsh	Taylor
Jane	Clark	Johnson	Marsh	Taylor
Julie	Clark	Johnson	Marsh	Taylor
Joan	Clark	Johnson	Marsh	Taylor

Determine the first and last name of each person.

1. If you were alphabetizing the names, the last first name and the last last name would go together.

2. Jane's and Julie's middle name is Ann. Joan's middle name is Lewis and Jean's is Lee.

3. Joan and Mrs. Johnson live on the same street.

4. One woman's initials spell out a word.

TARGET AREA 6: Logical Solutions   Situational Logic

*DIRECTIONS: A situation is described followed by a question. Mark the most logical solution from the three choices. See **CLUES** for help.*

1. John lives on the tenth floor in an apartment building. He is in the third grade and on school days he takes the elevator to the first floor. When he comes home after school, he takes the elevator to the seventh floor, then he walks up three flights of stairs. Why would he do this?

   ____ The elevator doesn't go up to the tenth floor.

   ____ He can only count up to seven, so that is the button he pushes.

   ____ He is too short to push the tenth-floor button; the seventh-floor button is as high as he can reach.

2. A wealthy father had a number of possessions to leave to his two daughters. He wanted his things divided equally between his daughters after he died. In order to do that, he thought of a solution that he felt would be fair. What would that solution be?

   ____ The daughters would gather all the things they both wanted and have them sold at auction. The one who bids the most would get them.

   ____ Each daughter would make a list of what she wanted. They would compare lists and circle the things they both wanted. They would discuss and bargain until they were both pleased with the outcome.

   ____ They would hire a lawyer who would randomly divide things equally between the two daughters.

3. A man in a restaurant found a dead fly in his coffee. He asked the waitress to bring him fresh coffee. She returned with another cup. When he took a sip from the new cup, he knew she had only removed the fly and not brought him a fresh cup of coffee. How could he know that?

____ The coffee was warm, not hot.

____ He had put sugar in his first cup before he noticed the fly, and this coffee also had sugar in it.

____ He knew the waitress was lying because she was not gone long enough to make a fresh cup of coffee.

---

4. A fierce-looking dog was chained to a tree in the front yard of a house. A delivery person wanted to go to the door, but he was afraid the dog would run and bite him. How best could he solve the problem?

____ He could throw the dog some food he had in his truck and hope it would be too busy eating to bother him.

____ He could walk around the tree several times out of reach of the dog. The dog would wind himself around the tree and not be able to get to the man as he went to the door.

____ The man could tell the dog to "sit" and "stay" before he walked to the door.

5. Jesse and Kelly are standing facing each other. They can talk to each other without raising their voices but they cannot see each other or touch each other. Why not?

_____ Jesse and Kelly are standing back to back on a sidewalk square.

_____ Jesse is standing on the bottom step, and Kelly is standing on the top step of a staircase.

_____ Jesse and Kelly are standing facing each other behind the same closed door.

---

6. For the last two years, Tom and Jerry have met at the same bar for martinis. Last Thursday was just the same. They each had a martini. They did not have any food or snacks. Tom downed his drink in three gulps and was fine. Jerry sipped his drink slowly and died a few hours later. The death was attributed somehow to the martini. What is the best explanation?

_____ Jerry choked on the olive in the martini.

_____ There was poison in the ice cubes in the glasses. Tom drank his drink before the ice had a chance to melt.

_____ Jerry was allergic to the grain used in the brand of vodka. Tom was not.

7. A man hung himself from a rope tied to a chandelier. When he was found, the room was empty except for the man hanging from the rope. Which explanation fits best as to how he died?

____ He swung the rope over the chandelier, put one end around his neck, and pulled himself up with the other end.

____ He really took pills to die; he just made it look like a hanging.

____ He turned up the heat in the room and stood on a block of ice that melted away.

8. A woman left her house and forgot her driver's license. Then she failed to obey a stop sign and went the wrong way down a one-way street. A policeman saw all this, but he did not arrest her. Why not?

____ The officer did not have any tickets with him.

____ She was walking, not driving.

____ These actions are not against the law in her state.

9. Mr. Smith and his son were involved in a bad car accident. Mr. Smith had minor injuries, but his son was seriously injured. In the hospital emergency center, the surgeon looked at the boy and said, "I can't operate on him, this is my son." How do you explain this?

____ The doctor had a son who could have been this boy's twin.

____ The doctor was not wearing his glasses and was wrong.

____ The doctor was the boy's mother.

10. Charlie was thrown in jail in a small remote town. He figured his only means of survival was to escape. He couldn't budge the cell bars and the door had multiple locks. The floor was packed earth. The walls of his cell were concrete and extended two feet into the ground and the ceiling was metal. There was one skylight just big enough to squeeze through if he could get to it. It was at least 15 feet high. He only had a small blanket to sit on, a metal bucket filled with water, and a small metal cup. Somehow he managed to escape. Which method makes the most sense?

_____ He banged on the bucket until someone came. He said he had had a dream that if he was not let out that a terrible storm would destroy the town. The townspeople were superstitious so they let him out.

_____ He dug holes around the sides of the cell and piled up the dirt below the skylight. Soon he could stand on the pile and reach the skylight.

_____ He used his cell phone to call his attorney. His attorney called the American Embassy, which paid his bail and sent a car to pick him up.

---

11. Sue was taking a walk when she witnessed a hit-and-run accident. She was able to see the six-digit license plate on the truck. She was carrying an umbrella and a book and nothing else. No one was around. Sue was able to give the numbers to the police hours later. What would have been the best way for Sue to remember? The license plate was: 134-857.

_____ She could tear out the book pages 1, 3, 4, 8, 5, and 7 and arrange them in that order.

_____ She could scratch the numbers into the grass with the end of the umbrella.

_____ She could fold over the tops of the book pages 13, 48, and 57.

Workbook for Cognitive Skills copyright © Susan Howell Brubaker 2009

12. A man was talking to a clerk at Home Depot. He asked the price of an item on display. The clerk said each item cost $2. The man asked if that would be $6 for 100. The clerk told him that was right. The man bought 84 and pays the clerk $4. How could this be correct?

____ Each item was a bag with many nails in it.

____ The items were on clearance sale.

____ Each item was a house number.

---

13. Rob was running toward home when he saw a masked man.
He stopped quickly, turned around, and began running back in the direction he had come from. Suddenly he deliberately slid to the ground and stayed there. Why?

____ Rob ran back to his wife who had stopped to pet a dog. He slid to the ground to put himself between the dog and his wife.

____ It was Halloween and the masked man was in costume. Rob slid on a candy wrapper and hurt his back.

____ Rob was playing baseball and running toward home base when he saw the catcher with the ball so he ran back to third base.

14. Liz was spending the winter with her daughter who lives in another state. She had a P.O. box and asked her neighbor Teresa to forward her mail. After Liz had not received any mail in two weeks, she called Teresa. Teresa told Liz that because she did not leave her with the key to the mailbox, she thought Liz had changed her mind. Liz apologized and said she would send Teresa the key. But Liz never did receive any mail from Teresa. What probably happened?

____ Teresa forgot she told Liz she would forward the letters.

____ Liz sent the key to her own address and the envelope with the key is still in her mailbox.

____ Teresa got the key and tried it but it didn't work on the box.

---

15. A mother told her children to do something, but only one boy obeyed. Then the woman said something to that boy that made him stomp away and go sulk in a corner. What is the best explanation of what happened?

____ The boy obeyed expecting to get money, but the mother didn't pay him so he got mad and stomped away.

____ The mother told the children that whoever wanted ice cream should go sit in a corner for five minutes.

____ They were all playing "Simon Says" and the boy did what she said but lost the game because the mother had not said "Simon Says."

16. An older man dressed all in black walked out in front of a car driven by a young driver. The driver had his headlights off and there were no streetlights. The driver was able to swerve just in time and avoid hitting the person. How come?

    ____ The man was almost seven feet tall, so the driver could see his face.

    ____ It was daytime, so the driver saw him in time to brake and avoid hitting him.

    ____ The driver really swerved to avoid a pothole in the road.

---

17. A gnat flew into my ear too deep for me to get it out. It started crawling and buzzing around inside my ear. I finally had an idea and was able to remove it. Which solution makes the most sense?

    ____ I put alcohol on a cotton pad and put it next to my ear. As the alcohol dried, it evaporated the gnat.

    ____ I blew my nose very hard and the gnat popped right out of my ear.

    ____ I put my ear down next to a bright lamp. The gnat was attracted by the light and flew out.

---

18. A passenger was really getting on the nerves of the taxi driver. The woman talked loudly and constantly. The driver wanted some peace and quiet. Since he had not said anything, he decided to pretend he was deaf and indicated that with gestures. It was a quiet ride. As the woman walked away from the cab at her destination, she suddenly realized the cab driver was not deaf. How did she know?

    ____ The driver said "thank you" when the woman handed him a tip.

    ____ The driver had to have heard her say where she wanted to be dropped off.

    ____ The driver spoke English to the next person who got in the cab.

TARGET AREA 6: Logical Solutions   Literal Meaning

DIRECTIONS: A situation is described followed by a question. Consider the information carefully before answering. The answer is logical but not always obvious. See CLUES for help.

1. Sam takes an hour and a half to run around a track when he goes in a clockwise direction. However, when he runs counterclockwise around the track, it takes him 90 minutes. How do you explain this?

   _____

2. How could you rewrite the following information so that it follows a pattern? May 6, 1978, at 12:34 p.m.

   _____

3. Mr. and Mrs. Smith have four sons. Each son has one sister. How many children are in the Smith family?

   _____

4. There are 12 one-cent stamps in a dozen. How many two-cent stamps are in a dozen?

   _____

5. How can you throw a tennis ball as hard as you can and have it come back to you without hitting a wall or anything else?

   _____

6. It takes ten minutes to boil water and make one hard-boiled egg. How many minutes would it take to make three eggs?

_____

7. A pig weighs 94 pounds when it is standing on three legs. How much would it weigh when standing on four legs?

_____

8. What are the three errors in the next sentence? Alan walked next door to visit his neighbor who just returned from Los Vegas.

_____

9. Two college kids decided to drive from Boston to Detroit to visit a friend. The trip took 14 hours, which they made in one day by sharing the driving. They also made the entire trip with a flat tire that they did not bother to fix. How could they do this?

_____

10. Since the millennium year of 2000, how many times have Christmas and New Year's Day fallen in the same year?

_____

11. Before Mt. Everest was discovered, what was the highest mountain range on Earth?

_____

12. What is it that happens twice in each moment, once in every minute, but never in a thousand years?

_____

13. Mary's mother has four children. The first child's name is April. The second child's name is May. The third child is June. What is the name of the fourth child?

_____

14. 1990 dollar bills are worth more than 1985 dollar bills. How much more and why?

_____

15. Name three consecutive days without using these words: Monday, Tuesday, Wednesday, Thursday, Friday, Saturday, or Sunday.

_____

16. Steve was in a pet shop looking at a parrot. The shop owner said, "I guarantee this bird will repeat every word it hears." Steve was impressed and bought the parrot. At his home, the bird would not repeat anything. Steve took it back to the pet shop and demanded his money back. The owner insisted he had not told a lie, and he would not give Steve a refund. What could be the explanation for this?

_____

17. In order to become president of the United States, a person must meet five requirements. He or she must be at least 35 years old. He or she must have been born in the United States. He or she must be a citizen and must have resided in the States for at least 14 years. What is the fifth and last requirement?

_____

18. Art took his dog for a walk one evening. About halfway through the walk, it started to rain. Art didn't have an umbrella and he was not wearing a hat. His clothes got soaked, the dog got wet, but not a hair on Art's head got wet. How could that be?

_____

19. Name the food that fits this description. You throw away the outside and cook the inside. Then you eat the outside and throw away the inside.

_____

TARGET AREA 6: Logical Solutions   Tricky Questions

DIRECTIONS: Read and consider the situation carefully before answering. The answers are
tricky, but will seem obvious if you think about them. See **CLUES** *for help.*

1. If the vice president of the United States died, who would become the president?

_____

2. You are the engineer of a train that goes from Denver to Chicago. The train trip covers 600 miles at an average speed of 85 miles per hour. The train leaves Denver at 6:00 p.m. What is the name of the engineer?

_____

3. I bought eight ears of corn and four tomatoes. For dinner, we ate everything but two ears of corn and one tomato. How much corn was left?

_____

4. You dig a hole that is two feet deep, two feet wide, and two feet long. How many feet of dirt are in the hole?

_____

5. You find an aladdin's lamp and a genie pops out and says he will grant you three wishes. What can you wish for to get the most from your three wishes?

_____

6. A gentleman went to an antique dealer to have two old books appraised that had been handed down in his family. One was a first edition autobiography of Robinson Crusoe. The second was a Nancy Drew mystery in its original jacket that was signed and dated by Nancy Drew. Were they valuable? Why or why not?

_____

7. Let's say an airplane full of people crashed right on the border of the United States and Canada. Where would the survivors be buried?

_____

8. Two people in the same family are sitting next to each other on a couch. The person on the left is the father of the person on the right. However, the person on the right is not his son. Who is the person on the right?

_____

9. How many letters of the alphabet can be written upside down?

_____

10. Ed travels 35 miles every day to his Chicago job. He does not use a plane, car, taxi, bus, subway, or anything else on wheels. He does not pass over water, sidewalks, streets, or use an animal. What could his job be?

_____

11. Two men played checkers for three hours. Each man played five games. Each man also won four games. How can this be?

_____

12. Jim sold Sam a radio for 60 dollars. Sam gave Jim a 50-dollar bill. How much change does Sam get?

_____

13. A murderer is condemned to death. He must enter one of three rooms. The first room is full of fire. The second one is full of assassins with loaded guns. The third room is full of lions that haven't eaten in two years. Which room should he choose and why?

_____

14. The year is 1958. Walter and his wife go to the movies. Walter strangles and kills his wife during the movie. He takes her back home with no one knowing what he has done. How could that happen?

_____

15. Mr. Smith owns a rooster. If it wanders over to Mr. Brown's yard and lays an egg, who owns the egg?

_____

16. Alex, Chris, and Sam sat in a bar and drank beer all night, but Alex and Sam never went to the men's room. Why not?

_____

17. The numbers 7 and 11 are both odd. Without adding, subtracting, multiplying or dividing, how can you make both numbers even?

_____

18. Two boys were born on the same day at the same time and to the same mother, but they were not twins. Why not?

_____

19. This item is black when you buy it, it is red when you use it, and it is gray when you throw it away. What could it be?

_____

20. The jury condemned Mr. Grant to death. The judge gave him some leniency and told him he could choose how he would die. What answer should he choose for a long life?

_____

CLUES

CLUES

Page 19, 20, 21: Missing One Letter, Missing Two Letters, Missing Three Letters

First answer: Page 19 – land,   Page 20 – cedar,   Page 21 – anthem

Clues: One of the words from each question is listed in scrambled order.

guitar	wire	eleven	clam	troop	operas
coast	booth	castle	agency	pill	slob
weave	load	flame	joke	each	bump

Page 22, 23: Shared Letters

First answer: the letter **D** (dim, Fred, code)

Clues: The shared missing letters are listed in alphabetical order. Letters may be repeated.

    a   c   e   i   l   n   o   p   r   s   t   u   v   y

Pages 24, 25, 26: Three-Word Titles

First answer: James Earl Jones

Clues: The initials of each item are listed in order reading across.

KAJ	GWC	YSL	MLK	HRC	FLW	EAP
CCM	ORC	KLP	AFC	SPS	CBH	VIC
TSS	ICS	BNB	WOF	TOF	MTP	ILL
LAO	SNL	ELR	PIR	AMC	GMA	

Pages 27, 28: Word Completion

First answer: armrest

Clues: The names that are formed are listed in scrambled order.

Michelle	Sue	Jennifer	Robert	Barb	Gerry / Terry
George	William	Jean	Tim	James	Carolyn

Pages 29, 30, 31, 32: Joined Words, Word Halves

First answer: Page 29 – anthem,   Page 31 – empire

Clues: The words for both exercises are listed in alphabetical order.

aboard	absolute	activity	archer	ashore	automate
baboon	bachelor	blockade	bounce	browsing	budget
button	chapel	charcoal	daffodil	errand	familiar
feathers	gemstone	generate	gravel	humidity	hybrid
income	juvenile	laughing	lipstick	liquid	mackerel
mahogany	margin	massacre	menace	moderate	monotone
mustache	normal	obtain	office	ourselves	palate
paradise	patron	physical	pleasure	portable	previous
reappear	restrain	romantic	rotate	routines	salary
season	shedding	squabble	starve	stubborn	truthful
twenty					

Pages 33, 34, 35, 36: Inserted Words, Interwoven Words

First answer: Page 33 – positive,   Page 35 – splint

Clues: The answers for both exercises are listed in alphabetical order.

adventure	bread	breath	business	calendar	chain
changed	count	crunch	drawer	establish	flamboyant
freedom	ghost	grateful	gravy	guidelines	hoarse
impatient	industry	island	locust	loneliness	lookout
meringue	mound	nutcracker	ornament	parrot	patient
plumb	president	problem	protect	pursue	rehearsal
resident	resource	scent	schooner	shampoo	sidewalk
smother	something	splice	strong	stubborn	support
telegram	trample	unfold	upholster	upkeep	vocabulary
weekend	wrestle	wring			

Pages 37, 38: Embedded Words

First answer: snowplow

Clues: The answers are listed in alphabetical order.

armadillo	bartender	breadbasket	candleholder	clothespin
coincidence	combination	commandment	cupboard	doorbell
earthworm	fellowship	hairbrush	hamburger	investigate
knowledge	Manhattan	parachute	photocopy	publicity
resignation	satisfaction	scarecrow	seventeen	shoestring
thermometer	tragically	wallflower	withdrawn	

Pages 39, 40: Heard Words

First answer: escort

Clues: The answers are listed in alphabetical order.

able	army	arrow	article	baby	begun	believe
blue jay	brandy	cedar	croquet	debate	duty	elsewhere
emotion	engine	explain	eyesight	fancy	fuel	gallon
harem	hazy	heiress	lazy	obey	people	prairie
season						

Pages 41, 42: Piggyback Words

First answer: notebook,   bookends

Clues: There are several possible answers. Our set of answers is listed in alphabetical order.

Words that start a compound word (column 1)

arm	bare	black	blank	chair	down	foul
frying	good	make	may	net	news	out
queen	quick	rough	scratch	second	to	time
turn	upside	watch				

Words that end a compound word (Column 2)

bone	book	cake	clothes	cutter	guest	hall
hills	hind	hunt	lash	law	lift	light
mare	off	paper	payment	shake	sides	spread
ways	whelm	wright				

Pages 43, 44: Compound Words

First answer: headquarters

Clues: There are several possible answers. Our set of answers is listed in alphabetical order.

ache	away	berry	bill	board	breathing	burn
burner	candle	cheese	collar	court	crystal	dial
day	diving	elbow	emery	eye	family	fill
fire	flash	flower	glasses	golf	great	hair
high	ironing	jay	ladies'	lights	master	moth
ordered	over	phones	pilot	red	ribbon	rise
screen	sky	sounding	start	sun	wrecking	

Page 45: Letter Addition

First answer: ate

Clues: There are several possible answers. Our set of possible answers is listed in scrambled order.

new	gem	eel	see	are	tea	eye
hey	rag	use	eat	red	ewe	one
yet	ear	age				

Pages 46, 47, 48: Category Crosswords

First answer: gray

Clues: Possible words for all the crosswords are listed in alphabetical order.

Reminder: Each page starts a new category.

apple	beer	blue	birch / beech	black	brown
cherry	cocoa	coffee	elm	espresso	juice
lemon	lemonade	magnolia	maple	milk	milkshake
oak	orange	palm	pink	poplar	red
sequoia	tea	walnut	water	white	willow
wine	yellow				

Page 49, 50, 51: Crossword Fill-Ins

First answer: The top three-letter word going down can be any three-letter word ending in **E**.

Clues: There are many possibilities. Our set of answers is listed alphabetically by the length of the word.

2- and 3-letter words

art	beg	car	egg	end	hot	in	let	nap
new	now	odd	one	or	row	sad	she	sir
sky	so	to	too	van				

4-letter words

bolt	boss	bugs	bush	clip	fact	file
hero	hold	itch	kick	lost	miss	nose
once	ring	riot	tree	week	when	yard

5- and 6-letter words

basket	dress	earth	gears	horns	never	noisy
pansy	rates	ready	start	tease	twelve	whole

Pages 52, 53: Mini-Grids

First answer: One set of words for the first grid could be: **the** and **try**.

Clues: There are a number of possible answers. Our set of answers is listed in alphabetical order. The across words have an asterisk (*).

Page 52

arm	ask	ate*	bed	box*	bus*	cat*	cup	dry*
ego	elf*	fad	fly	gas	her	hum	ice*	jar*
job	law*	map	mix	old*	owl	pen*	rag*	rib
sun*	tin	toe	use*	web*	wet			

Page 53

able*	ace	back*	bat	bath	cell*	chew
cut	damp	dark	dove	drag*	fair*	fry
game	harm*	herb*	howl*	inch	iron*	jazz*
kept	key	kind*	knee*	low	nail	quit
rib	run	smog*	stub*	thaw*	tidy*	tie
tile*	trap*	unit*	urge	used	west*	yawn*

Page 54, 55: Crossword Grids

First Answer: Page 54 – Using this set of answers, the top word across is **plot**. Page 55 – Using this set of answers, the top word across is **lunch**.

Clues: There are a number of possible answers for each puzzle. Our set of answers is listed alphabetically by length of the word.

as	so	to	all	awe	get	gym	ice
ink	lid	new	old	own	rug	dump	envy
grab	lake	long	moth	plot	send	spin	turn
adult	ashes	exact	favor	lunch	either		

Page 59, 60, 61, 62, 63, 64, 65, 66, 67: Related Matches

First Answer: run

Clues: For each page, the first letter of each answer is listed in order.

Page 59: k, s, m, e, v, o, t, b, s   **Page 60:** e, a, t, p, m, b, t, f, d, s

Page 61: s, h, b, a, s, b, r, t, a, a   **Page 62:** s, g, b, i, a, c, l, i, d, c

Page 63: p, a, n, c, e, v, i, c, f, c   **Page 64:** P, B, J, E, G, C, M, R, S, L

Page 65: w, b, d, s, l, b, b, m, f, s   **Page 66:** f, p, d, v, n, s, i, c, c, a

Page 67: r, h, c, c, d, l, f, h, a, p

Pages 68, 69: Overlapping Phrases

First answer: clean up your <u>room</u>,   <u>room</u> service

Clues: The answers are listed in alphabetical order.

age	better	box	check	come	day	down	easy
go	guest	home	know	life	look	luck	mind
more	order	out	party	please	right	room	run
shot	sleep	take	that	time	up		

Pages 70, 71, 72: Common Phrases

First answer: fame and fortune

Clues: The first letter of each answer is listed in order.

Page 70: h, d, n, f, p, t, r, p

Page 71: t, r, s, l, b, t, s, m, f, l, b, s

Page 72: h, g, t, r, l, d, f, l, n, r

Pages 73, 74, 75, 76, 77, 78: Alliterative Phrases, Alliterative Terms

First answer: Page 73 – rock and roll   Page 75 – baby boomer

Clues: For each exercise, the first word (or word part) of the answer is listed.

Pages 73 and 74

1. rock	2. black	3. spic	4. trick	5. wash	6. stars
7. do's	8. feast	9. now	10. drink	11. socks	12. tried
13. bed	14. rules	15. rags	16. bread	17. safe	

Pages 75, 76, 77, 78

2. beer	3. secondhand	4. bumble	5. match	6. belly	
7. cable	8. secret	9. community	10. cheese	11. french	
12. happy	13. leading	14. black	15. parcel	16. pet	
17. penny	18. marsh	19. sales	20. direct	21. sight	
22. money	23. social	24. stainless	25. sweat	26. Academy	
27. tongue	28. tow	29. vice	30. whole	31. hour	
32. play	33. bad	34. scared			

Pages 79, 80, 81, 82: Words in Common

First answer: overtime

Clues: The first letter of each missing word is listed.

1. o u a,   t y,   b s   2. n,   f,   a t,   g
3. w,   b,   p,   s t,   b p   4. o t,   p,   c,   w,   w
5. o a n l,   t a,   p,   t o c,   w y   6. o t m,   s,   c,   l,   o t l
7. c,   c,   e,   i u,   t i   8. d l,   s,   w,   I,   j

Page 83: Rhyming Words

First answer: prime time

Clues: The missing letters of the first word are listed.

2. H	3. bl	4. fl	5. n	6. a	7. f	8. p	9. b	
10. b	11. c	12. gr	13. w	14. ch	15. wh	16. tr		

Page 84, 85, 86: Clichés

First answer: spill the beans

Clues: The first letter of the missing word is listed.

Page 84

2. b	3. c	4. c	5. p	6. t	7. d	8. b
9. b	10. p	11. c	12. b	13. h	14. d	15. w
16. t	17. s	18. p			

Page 85

1. f	2. n	3. d	4. r	5. s	6. a	7. t
8. p	9. o	10. o	11. l	12. f	13. m	14. l
15. t	16. p	17. j	18. o	19. n	20. s

Page 86

1. c	2. d	3. a	4. c	5. d	6. m	7. e
8. s	9. f	10. w	11. g	12. b	13. w, s	14. c, m
15. l, l	16. g, c				

Page 87, 88: Category Phrases

First answer: bread

Clues: The answers are listed in alphabetical order.

apple	bill	bob	bull	cat	collar	face
foot	frog	gloves	gold	green	head	heart
horse	jack	lip	pants	red	shoe	slip
tea	toast	tom	white	yellow	

Pages 89, 90: Abbreviations to Words

First answer: RI (Rhode Island)

Clues: The abbreviations for both pages are listed in alphabetical order.

BA	CIA	COD	EST	FBI	GI	IOU
NBC	RIP	SE	TGIF	UN	USA	

Pages 91, 92: **Motivating Quotes**

First answer: Laughter is the . . .

Clues: The first two words of the quote are listed.

2. Don't give	7. Smile and	12. Tomorrow is	17. Look for
3. Nothing ventured	8. There are	13. Don't look	18. Where there's
4. You are	9. When one	14. Challenge is	19. Attitude and
5. Don't find	10. Count your	15. Winners never	20. A day
6. Life is	11. If you	16. Laugh and	

Pages 93, 94, 95: **Incomplete Proverbs**

First answer: An apple a day . . .

Clues: The first incomplete word is listed in each question.

2. count	7. judge	12. Nothing	17. People	22. fair
3. news	8. heads	13. took	18. Birds	23. bite
4. Honesty	9. grass	14. best	19. penny	
5. April	10. teach	15. early	20. Rome	
6. put	11. Actions	16. Absence	21. rolling	

Pages 96, 97: **Split Sayings**

First answer: There's no

Clues: The <u>second</u> word in each saying is listed.

2. sleeping	4. is	6. method	8. easier
3. in	5. hands	7. is	9. doesn't

Pages 98, 99, 100: Phrases to Grid

First Answer: The top word across in the top left grid is **no**.

Clues: The top words across in each grid are listed in scrambled order.

is	rose	together	better	for	deep
the	life	life	between	look	

Pages 101, 102: Completion Word Search

First answer: Anything is <u>possible</u>. POSSIBLE is hidden in the second row on the right.

Clues: The words to find in the grid are listed in scrambled order.

fragile	thousand	simple	salvation	mountain	dictionary
allegiance	warrant	matter	litter	nothing	chairman
facts	collar	dotted	behavior	defense	

Pages 103, 104, 105: Celebrity Links

First answer: TV news reporters

Clues: A short hint to their common fame is listed in scrambled order.

classical music	chef	country music	unsportsmanlike	boxing
nursery rhyme	model	cake	actress	movie
Shakespeare	Disney	product	rock music	politics
President	family	Bible	fashion	

Pages 106, 107, 108: Celebrity Descriptions

First answer: Tiger Woods

Clues: The initials of each celebrity are listed in alphabetical order by first name.

BF	BG	BO	CE	DC	DT	HH	JA
MLK	MS	NA	OW	PW	RR	VVG	WD

Pages 109, 110, 111: First Names

First answer: Jane

Clues: The first names are listed in alphabetical order.

Ben	Billy	Bob	Carol	Charles	Dennis	Donald
Dr.	Fred	George	Jennifer	Jerry	Jimmy	
John	Mary	Michael	Paul	Robert	Steven	

Pages 112, 113, 114: Last Names

First answer: Ford

Clues: The last names are listed in alphabetical order.

Allen	Brown	Bush	Cooper	Fox	Grant	Jackson
Jones	King	Marx	Rogers	Roosevelt	Simon	Simpson
Smith	Stewart	Turner	White	Williams		

Pages 115, 116: Incomplete Names

First answer: Bette

Clues: All of the names (first and last) are listed in alphabetical order.

Albert	Armstrong	Barbra	Barry	Berry	Beethoven
Bill	Bruce	Butler	Carey	Cruise	David
DeGeneres	Dion	Ernest	Frank	Franklin	Gandhi
Harry	Hoffman	Jack	James	John	Johnny
Johnson	Jolie	Jones	Katherine	Leonardo	Lincoln
Lou	Mark	Michael	Nicole	O'Brien	O'Neal
Philbin	Reagan	Richard	Rowlings	Ryan	Steele
Streep	Timberlake	Vader	Washington	Wayne	Winston
Wonder					

Pages 117, 118, 119: Literal Phrases

First answer: mixed messages

Clues: The answers are listed in alphabetical order reading down.

centerfold	growing pains	round of applause
check's in the mail	hit below the belt	safety in numbers
coffee break	hole in one	sleeping on the job
double park	life after death	take one at bedtime
down to earth	little fish in a big pond	two-car garage
foreign language	love at first sight	unfinished business
forever and a day	right between the eyes	wait on hand and foot
for sale	right in the middle of everything	you're under arrest

Pages 123, 124, 125, 126, 127, 128: Defined Times Two, Defined Times Three

First answer: Page 123 – miss,   Page 125 – ring

Clues: The answers are listed in alphabetical order.

bank	bar	bat	board	box	cast	club
cold	date	fast	file	fine	lean	mercury
nail	oil	pass	pitch	pool	pound	press
raise	rock	rolls	seal	store	tip	trunk
watch	well					

Pages 129, 130, 131: Alphabet Elimination

First answer: yesterday

Clues: The answers are listed in scrambled order.

jealous	subpoena	excellent	amethyst	question	squeeze
kindergarten	family	equator	volunteer	hilarious	expensive
cheeseburger	sterilize	before	lightning	next	brazil
candidate	banquet	perform	juice	woodpecker	beaver
intermediate	champion	jaywalk	waves		

Pages 132, 133, 134, 135: Overlapped Words

First answer: fast

Clues: The answers are listed in alphabetical order.

afraid	alto	aroma	arrest	awake	canada
celery	cellar	cello	charge	cheese	chocolate
church	dance	earth	eleven	envelope	explode
female	game	germany	idea	index	kennel
leash	least	lime	loaf	match	medicine
menu	necklace	new	nurse	opal	ounce
peach	petite	raw	recipe	red	rye
search	severe	short	stable	stare	stone
stop	tennis	termite	test	thin	tooth
year					

Pages 136, 137, 138: Missing Ends

First answer: shiver

Clues: The answers are listed in alphabetical order.

alien	ashes	bribe	champ	change	chase
crawl	drowsy	enamel	factory	frown	gate
hearse	heart	jewel	king	lamb	mask
mouth	obey	odor	panda	photo	planet
rodeo	scarf	scowl	steam	steel	stool
sweet	thumb	wages	wedges		

Pages 139, 140, 141, 142: Missing Middles

First answer: aloha

Clues: The answers are listed in scrambled order.

repair	eagle	kick	window	groundhog	medium
nightgown	america	plump	ticket	diamond	revolver
xerox	high	recliner	throat	newborn	yearly
ohio	scissors	bib	employee	fireproof	drowned
critic	widow	label	museum	success	

Pages 143, 144, 145, 146: Triple Letters

First answer: Australia

Clues: The answers are listed in scrambled order.

needle	trespass	highlight	cranberry	unusual
lollipop	fifty-five	eccentric	toothpaste	emergency
nineteen	invitation	tattoo	divided	monopoly
bobby	surrender	banana	imitation	expensive
powwow	giggle	exercise	bikini	puppy
maximum	daddy	nonsense	assist	

Pages 147, 148: Word Plus Letter

First answer: parade

Clues: The first two letters of each answer are listed.

2. ab	3. re	4. pa	5. el	6. Fr	7. wa
8. mi	9. st	10. st	11. li	12. in	13. ra
14. bo	15. ti	16. mo	17. mo		

Pages 149, 150: Scrambled Triplets

First answer: dollar

Clues: The answers are listed in scrambled order.

scorch	murder	buckle	eraser	cereal
pencil	retire	exhale	muffin	wicked
hornet	orange	maroon	rescue	scream
period	shrink	voyage	drapes	police
oxygen	remove	twelve	forget	garage

Pages 151: Double Meanings

First answer: blue

Clues: The answers are listed in alphabetical order.

bowls	date	glasses	green	lemon
mugs	orange	pants	pitcher	prune
rose	slip	sock	tan	tie

Pages 152, 153: Fractured Words

First answer: French toast

Clues: The first words on each line are listed in alphabetical order.

Apple	Baked	Baltimore	Boston	Chicago	Chocolate
Denver	Detroit	Honolulu	Indianapolis	Milwaukee	Nashville
Orlando	Peanut	Philadelphia	Pickle	Portland	Pumpkin
Salad	Seattle	Shredded	Strawberry	Topeka	

Pages 154, 155: Letter Removal

First answer: smother, mother   The letter on the line is <u>M</u>

Clues: The words with clues are listed in scrambled order.

neat	pine	steam	room	bait	wed	hoe
end	stem	lend	brake	want	owed	knight
drugs	pin	pane	lawns	broom	ant	parka
home	stink	thin	car	park	night	below
laws	scar	net	pad	bake	paid	sink
bat	rugs	blow	plane	think		

Pages 156, 157, 158, 159, 160, 161: Letter Transfers

First answer: pay

Clues: The answers to the definitions are listed alphabetically in order of length.

end	hay	sue	war	coat	coke	diet
dirt	golf	less	maps	suit	teen	tied
yams	album	beast	built	chase	fight	least
meals	month	rinse	satin	seven	smile	stamp
teeth	thigh	unite	advice	afghan	apples	banana
cotton	demand	eighty	higher	street	tomato	gondola
hatchet	luggage	station	thought	chapters	governor	

Pages 162, 163: Building Words

First Answer: The final answer of the first question is **twine**.

Clues: The final answers are listed in alphabetical order. Subtract one letter and work back to the beginning to get all words.

breast	flash	marine	party	stone

Pages 164, 165, 166: Word Addition

First answer: me

Clues: The first word (and first part of the final answer) in each item is listed.

2. wheel	3. bad	4. pen	5. out	6. term
7. but	8. new	9. to	10. car	11. Dan

Pages 167, 168, 169: Word Splits

First answer: airport

Clues: The longest word in each item is listed in alphabetical order.

acrobat   bathroom   collide   contest   bracelet   faith   friend

manager   number   ornament   parakeet   promises   tornado

Pages 170, 171: Chained Words

First answer: cab + I + net = cabinet

Clues: The first word in each item is listed.

2. me	3. big	4. cat	5. cent	6. bob	7. her
8. leg	9. tom	10. connect	11. mar	12. inn	13. art
14. barb	15. pan	16. ant	17. on		

Pages 172, 173: Changing Phrases

First answer: (tabby) cat

Clues: The answers are listed in scrambled order.

bug	can	hat	law	pack	pole	Sam
hen	Tim	man	park	saw	toe	car
Rock	hog	mat	pen	role	sea	top
hole	Tom	mug	dog	dam	tub	wet
pet	hose	roll	jaw	net	pie	den
rub	sock	pin	rug	sack	tea	hot
nut	tie	dot	set	pit	not	web

Pages 174, 175, 176: Rhyming Phrases

First answer: nickel pickle

Clues: The first word of each item is listed.

2. big	3. sad	4. cheap	5. late	6. real	7. best
8. great	9. rare	10. funny	11. weird	12. good	
13. fine	14. hound	15. brain	16. your	17. spare	
18. drill	19. guest	20. old	21. junk	22. chief	

Pages 179, 180: Omitted Letter

First answer: earn, lean

Clues: Cover one letter at a time in each word to see which combination makes a new word.

Pages 181, 182: Disguised Words

First answer: towel

Clues: The answers are listed in scrambled order.

nail	flooding	crab	letter	cream	dress	gold
pin	scale	beaver	robe	sleet	card	haddock
coat	dart	trout	sink	sword	wind chill	tiger
green	novel	tan	paper	sheep	storm	moose
comb	vest	warm	tie	pants	shark	black
perch	shoes	gray	pills	saw	bass	book
snow	goat	tuna	fork	bear	fog	rain
soap	bull	note	star	pen	pink	

Pages 183, 184, 185, 186: Scrambled Words

First answer: post

Clues: The first letter in each word is listed.

1. p, t, S   2. s, t, b   3. a, m, n   4. d, k, s
5. d, e, t   6. c, c, t   7. e, t, t   8. b, b, r
9. s, s, l   10. b, b, b   11. d, d, p   12. p, p, p
13. m, s, t   14. g, g, d   15. s, p, s   16. p, p, p

Pages 187, 188: Word Reversals

First answer: plug, gulp

Clues: The answers are listed in alphabetical order.

bats	don	drawer	flow	guns	keep	net
nod	pals	part	paws	peek	pots	rat
raw	reward	slap	snug	stab	stop	swap
tar	ten	trap	war	wolf		

Pages 189, 190, 191, 192, 193: Specific Letters

First answer: accept

Clues: The answers for these pages are listed in alphabetical order reading down.

AFFLUENT	EXECUTIVE	JOKING	PRIVATE	UNEATEN
AGAIN	EXPLOSION	JOURNAL	PROBLEM	UNLESS
AMUSE	FARM	KNEAD	PROUD	URGE
BAPTIZE	FAVOR	KNOT	QUACK	VALLEY
BAZAAR	FLAKE	KNOWN	QUAIL	VALUE
BLANK	FLAMINGO	KNUCKLE	QUARTER	VARIETY
BOXER	FLOWERS	LACQUER	QUARTZ	VICTORY
BRANCH	FLUID	LAWYER	QUILT	VOCABULARY
BUCKET	FORMAL	LIBERTY	RAINBOW	WALRUS
CAMPAIGN	FOXES	LOGIC	RAISE	WHEEL
CANDLE	GENTLE	LONELY	REJECT	WIZARD
CASHEW	GHOST	MANUAL	REVIEW	WORSE
CAVITY	GOPHER	MATRIMONY	SCENT	X-RAY
CHIEF	GROAN	MEDICAL	SCOLD	XYLOPHONE
CLOVER	GROUCH	MEMBER	SHAVE	YANKEE
COMEDY	HALF	MOIST	SMOOTH	YAWNING
CRATER	HAZARD	NARROW	SPOIL	YEAST
CURFEW	HEARTH	NEPHEW	SQUASH	YIELD
DAIRY	HEAVY	NERVOUS	SUBJECT	YOUTH
DAMP	HEDGEHOG	NIGHT	SUEDE	ZEBRA
DIAGRAM	HOWL	NOVEL	THEATER	ZERO
DISTANT	IDEAL	OATMEAL	THICK	ZEST
DRIVER	INDUSTRY	OBJECT	TICKLE	
ENJOY	INHERIT	OFFER	TROPHY	
EQUALITY	INQUIRE	PELICAN	TULIP	
ERRAND	JERSEY	PRICE	UMPIRE	

Workbook for Cognitive Skills copyright © Susan Howell Brubaker 2009

Pages 194, 195, 196: Repeated Letters

First answer: FIFTH

Clues: The answers for the pages are listed in alphabetical order going across.

ADVANTAGE	AMMONIA	ANTENNA	ANYBODY	ARTIFICIAL
ATTEMPT	ATTRACTIVE	BELIEVE	BALLERINA	BIKINI
BREATHE	BUBBLES	BUMBLEBEE	CABOOSE	CANADA
COCKROACH	COCOON	CORPORATION	DAFFODIL	DANDRUFF
DEDICATED	DISASTER	DIVIDED	DRESSES	EGGNOG
ELECTRIC	ETIQUETTE	FISHHOOK	FLANNEL	FLUFFY
FOSSIL	FREEZER	GARBAGE	GOSSIP	HAPPINESS
HAWAIIAN	HEADACHE	HICCUPS	HIGHLIGHT	HOSTESS
HUMOROUS	ICING	IMMATURE	JIGGLE	KHAKI
LADDER	MADAM	MANNEQUIN	MATINEE	MAXIMUM
MIDDLE	MIRROR	MORNING	MOTOR	PARADE
PARALLEL	PEOPLE	PEPPERMINT	PINEAPPLE	PIONEER
PIZZA	POWWOW	QUARREL	SCRIBBLE	SNEEZE
SUBURBAN	SURRENDER	SWEET	TIPTOE	TOBACCO
TREATMENT	UNDERSTANDING	UNUSUAL	VACUUM	VELVET
WINDOW	XEROX	ZUCCHINI		

Pages 197, 198: Multiple Missing Letters

First answer: hardware

Clues: The answers are listed in alphabetical order.

adult	anxiety	apologize	ballot	basket	beyond
blazer	cinnamon	coconut	comfort	crazy	crumble
dozen	equator	exhale	exotic	finally	foreign
forever	freckles	graph	growl	hammock	husband
imagine	inflation	injury	jogging	kitchen	lavender
leather	leaves	library	lobster	lukewarm	majority
masquerade	multiply	mustard	nightmare	nursery	objective
olives	orchid	painter	peanut	physical	preview
promotion	qualify	quickly	sixteen	soldier	standard
substance	teaspoon	unhappy	uniform	weakness	wedge
welcome					

Pages 199, 200: Consecutive Letters

First answer: cabbage

Clues: The answers for the pages are listed in alphabetical order.

abduct	abundance	almond	assault	back	buckled
canopy	champion	clothing	code	confirm	cultivate
cupboard	decay	defend	interesting	drastic	drawback
dust	edifice	education	evaluate	fabric	fighter
folder	forget	golfed	grief	hinge	hustle
lonesome	mental	manuscript	money	normal	November
ornament	piano	refrigerator	sliced	slight	strange
supportive	termites	unopened	vault	weigh	

First answer: acceptance

Clues: The answers are listed in alphabetical order.

bedspread	caterpillar	drawbridge	especially	fashionable
fortunate	guarantee	harmonica	interrupt	jeopardy
kindness	lifeguard	meditate	newspaper	outstanding
paralyze	quicksand	rectangle	sympathetic	telegram
volcano	wardrobe			

Pages 203, 204: Double Insertions

First answer: imitate

Clues: The first three letters of each answer are listed.

2. che	3. aba	4. fol	5. bar	6. ded	7. gar
8. lan	9. imp	10. mis	11. quo	12. swa	13. off
14. hin	15. roo	16. rai	17. ban	18. fif	19. ten
20. hap	21. nor	22. tho	23. viv	24. alc	25. unf
26. pol	27. slu	28. zuc	29. tra	30. yes	

Pages 205, 206: Letter Pairs

First answer: ou (courageous)

Clues: The first three letters of each answer are listed.

1. phi,   alf,   tre,   mam
2. dis,   non,   hea,   taf,   pic
3. por,   acc,   mar,   fur,   pri,   bar
4. sau,   emb,   beg,   leg,   hor,   pos
5. oin,   lic,   abs,   alu,   res,   fra

Pages 207, 208: Word Transformation

First Answer: The second line answer goes from PAPER to MANER.

Clues: The answer word is related in some way to the word you start with.

Page 207: 1. The answer is **money**.   2. The answer is **organ**.

Page 208: 3. The answer is **ice cream**.   4. The answer is **apple**.

Pages 209, 210: Word Construction

First Answer: POSTPONE is the first word.

Clues: Transfer any letters you can down or up to the next line. The first and last words are listed.

Page 209: **CRACKERS** is the last word.

Page 210: **DRESSING** is the first word. **MARYLAND** is the last word.

Pages 211, 212: Word Rebuses

First answer: Many

Clues: All of the answers are listed alphabetically by length of word.

a	is	to	cat	one	way
you	leap	look	make	more	skin
than	work	hands	light	there	before

Pages 213, 214: Word Squares

First Answer: One across and **one down** need to start with the same letter, so the word is **bars**.

Clues: A word from each puzzle is listed. Look for boxes in which the letters need to be the same.

In the second puzzle, the **one across** word is **star**.

In the third puzzle, the **one across** word is **word**.

Pages 216, 217, 218, 219, 220: **Letter Fill-Ins**

First answer: Using this set of answers, the first word across on page 216 is **assist**. The top word across on page 217 is **life**. The top word across on page 218 is **dough**.

Clues: There are a number of possible answers for each crossword. One set of possible answers is listed alphabetically by length of word.

Pages 216, 217, 218

go	it	me	or	up	ask	hen
led	oil	try	why	born	dark	echo
feet	fold	here	life	love	quit	rust
solo	well	actor	album	below	dough	grass
later	pilot	smash	spoon	steer	toast	upset
assist	bakery	corner	escape	filthy	gadget	gravel
growth	luxury	refill	string	throat	walnut	trophy
unique	archery	brother	curious	diploma	journal	machine
message	officer	pajamas	perfect	quietly	romance	rooster
rowboat	seasick	sterile	thirsty	volcano	worried	wrapper
yawning						

Pages 219, 220

am	my	so	gym	ill	may	use
acre	chef	code	inch	lion	moth	once
seam	sigh	walk	wasp	yard	agent	beach
elbow	fault	flirt	giant	glass	green	heavy
kneel	ledge	mauve	niece	novel	ounce	relax
shrub	sting	style	tulip	twist	absent	almond
anchor	arctic	banana	behind	career	debate	editor
ginger	lawyer	lilacs	murder	oblong	orchid	peanut
police	prefer	quench	reduce	refill	swerve	yellow
academy	captain	collect	contest	dentist	extinct	fatigue
formula	longest	muffler	musical	neutral	nothing	project
register	slender	symptom	therapy	traffic	vampire	specific

First Answer: One side of the die does not have any black spots on it.

Clue: The question about each picture suggests the part of the picture that is missing.

1. What is on all sides of a die?
2. How do you shoot it?
3. What?? What??
4. How do you put it in a purse?
5. How do you play it?
6. How do you close it?
7. How is the ride?
8. How does the water get in?
9. How does it walk?
10. What happens after dark?
11. How many directions are there?
12. How would you talk or eat?
13. Where do you blow?
14. How do you get the milk?

| Pages 225, 226, 227: | Picture Descriptions |

First answer: 9, rose

Clues: The names of the pictures as well as the answers are listed.

Page 225: The pictures represent: snowman, whistle, hair, star, rainbow, bells, four-leaf clover, eyes, rose, and anchors. The answers in order are: 9, 6, 5, 1, 7, 3, 10, 2, 4, 8

Page 226: The pictures represent: gun, king, roof, pond, cat, foot, star, grapes, bird, and shark. The answers in order are: 15, 12, 19, 17, 20, 14, 16, 11, 18, 13

Page 227: The pictures are: collar, basket, sun, button, bed, nickels, well, pants, beach ball, and bread. The answers in order are: 30, 22, 28, 24, 26, 21, 25, 23, 27, 29

Pages 228, 229, 230: Visual Compounds

First answer: collarbone–the first picture on the left (collar) with the sixth one on the right (bone)

Clues: The names of each picture are listed in order.

Page 228

collar	ear	flower	butter	sun	table	candle
pot	glasses	sticks	fly	ring	bone	spoon

Page 229

bed	cork	fire	note	shoe	turtle	wheel
hand	horn	pan	book	neck	chair	screw
gun	cracker					

Page 230

basket	cup	door	finger	sun	check	tooth
watch	bell	book	dog	ball	nail	brush
cake	flower					

Pages 231, 232, 233, 234, 235, 236, 237: Picture Elimination

First Answer: picture 6 (the eyes are open, full beard, and not wearing a suit)

Clues: Read carefully. The number of the correct picture on each page is listed.

Page 232: picture 5   **Page 233:** picture 4   **Page 234:** picture 1

Page 235: picture 2   **Page 236:** picture 3   **Page 237:** picture 2

Pages 238, 239: Letters in Common

First Answer: the letter c (all the words have **C** in them)

Clues: The first letter in each item is listed.

2. h   3. p   4. s

Pages 240, 241: Spoonerisms

First answer: <u>faded sheet</u> goes with <u>shaded feet</u> (number 4). The places of <u>f</u> and <u>sh</u> are switched.

Clues: The first match in each item is listed.

Page 241: <u>tot scale</u> goes with <u>Scot tale</u>. The places of <u>t</u> and <u>sc</u> are switched.

<u>change street</u> goes with <u>strange cheat</u>. The places of <u>ch</u> and <u>str</u> are switched.

Pages 242, 243: Letter Logic

First Answer: The letter **L** is not in goof.

Clues: The first letter in each item is listed.

2. The letter **E** is not in full.

3. The letter **G** is not in tear.

4. The letter **P** is not in ache.

Pages 244, 245: Word Characteristics

First answer: The first answer is GIGGLE.

Clues: The first letters of the answers in order are listed.

P, U, F, K, T, S, C, D, E, C, B, M, S, T

Pages 246, 247: Multiple Errors

First Answer: Starting at the top left corner, the years 2007 and 2012 at the right do not match.

Clues: It will help to scan the pictures from top to bottom or right to left as you look for errors.

Page 246: There are 10 intentional errors on the calendar.

Page 247: Starting on the top line, SAND WITCHES should be spelled **SANDWICHES**.

There are 36 intentional errors on the menu. You may find more or less depending on whether you judge some food prices as too high or too low.

Pages 248, 249, 250: Hidden Words

First Answer: The first three words that start with **A** are: as, ash, ashore

Clues: Use the strategy of starting with the first letter and find as many words as you can that start with that letter before moving to the next letter. The first three words in each item are listed.

2. pa, pan, pant, panther

3. bra, brace, bracelet

4. tea, teas, tease

5. bad, badminton, ad

6. at, attack, tack

7. me, medal, medallion

8. pa, page, age

Pages 251, 252, 253, 254: Letter Blocks

First answer: Line 1 goes into the 3rd box down. The hidden word in the white box is WALTZ.

Clues: The hidden words are listed in alphabetical order by page.

<u>**Page 251**</u>: comic, erase, point, satin, sting, waltz

<u>**Page 252**</u>: among, basic, flash, ideal, joker, level, north, relax, under, vinyl

<u>**Page 253**</u>: awake, chair, early, gravy, human, learn, lobby, mixer, quart, tribe

<u>**Page 254**</u>: actor, child, fifth, force, jelly, lodge, music, ready, snarl, young

---

Pages 255, 256: Defined Numbers

First Answer: 5 toes on one foot

Clues: The answers are listed in chronological order. A few numbers are used more than once.

1, 2, 3, 4, 5, 6, 7, 8, 9, 10, 11, XII, 13, 14, 18, 20, 24, 26, 29, 30, 32, 40, 50, 52, 365, 1,000

Page 257: Crossword Math

First answer: The answer to **1 across** is **365**

Clues: All of the answers to complete the puzzle are listed in chronological order.

11, 13, 21, 25, 28, 31, 32, 33, 39, 50, 52, 66, 83, 103, 360, 500

Pages 258, 259, 260: Word Searches

First Answer: EASY

Clues: The words to find in the grid are listed as they appear in the book. The words are written as you would find see them in the grid.

Page 258

BELTS	TOSS	RELY	ABOUT	DOZE
KENNEL	HAIR	CATCH	FLY	SEW
MOON	BEWARE	FORK	NUT	USED

Page 259

ASSOC	FEB	NW
AVE	HWY	PKG
BLDG	JR	LB
CAPT	MISC	RR
ETC	MT	TUES

ARIZONA	FLORIDA	ILLINOIS	NEWYORK
COLORADO	GEORGIA	KENTUCKY	TEXAS

Page 260

ALL →	C → PALATE	BUCKLE ↑	COUNT ↓
CIVIL →S	→ FIELD	C ↑ CAKE	↓ POUR
F → EN	→ HANDED	MAKE ↑	↓ TOWN
→ ANGLE	→ OVERS	↑ SET	LIE ↓
→ OFWAY	→ TURN	↑ SIDE ↓	TOUCH↓

Page 261, 262: Word Fill-Ins

First Answer: The first word down at the top left with the third letter O is **SPOT**.

Clues: You will sometimes need to compare the third or fourth letters to find the correct word. Two words on each page are listed.

<u>**Page 261:**</u> The bottom word reading across beginning with **Y** is **YOUR**.

<u>**Page 262:**</u> The first word reading down at the top left is **DECAF**.

The bottom word reading across with the second letter U is **MUFFIN**.

Pages 265, 266, 267, 268: Context Clues

First answer: coffee

Clues: The answers are listed in alphabetical order.

brain	candles	chocolate	collar	cough
envelope	grass	jeans	mirror	slippers

Pages 269, 270: Letter Words

First answer: I owe you for the peas.

Clues: The first two words are spelled out correctly.

2. I see	5. I see	8. You are	11. I am
3. Jay is	6. Are you	9. Ours is	12. I ate
4. I am	7. Alex owes	10. Seize the	13. Tennis is

Pages 271, 272: Homonym Sentences

First answer: I'll buy

Clues: The first two words are spelled out correctly.

2. For sale:	6. The knight	10. We tracked	14. Please choose
3. Our son	7. I knew	11. Their cruise	15. I guessed
4. I owe	8. Aunt Jeannie	12. Hugh's aunt	16. Please tighten
5. Do not	9. I told	13. I heard	17. Which one

Pages 273, 274: Unusual Definitions

First Answer: hijack (Hi, Jack)

Clues: The first two answers on each page are listed.

Page 273: 2. minimum (mini mum)

Page 274: 1. rebellion (rebel lion)   2. everest (Eve rest)

Pages 275, 276: Word Similarities

First answer: Each word has double letters in it.

Clues: Hints to the answers are listed in scrambled order.

first and last letters	rhyming words	same 4 letters
words are names	triple vowels	alphabetical order
compound words	Y = only vowel	add a letter
triple consonants	reads both ways	2 letters = 4-letter word
sounds like the letters		

Pages 277, 278, 279: Calendar Dates

First answer: 19th

Clues: There are five correct answer dates <u>and</u> six wrong dates listed below.

4   7   9   12   13   16   21   23   27   29   30

Pages 280, 281, 282, 283: Letter Tracking, Directional Words

First answer: Page 280 – copy   Page 282 – barn

Clues: The word that is formed in each item is listed in alphabetical order.

along	danger	dragon	frugal
grind	hedge	noting	yard

First Answer: acre

Clues: Note the page numbers for the answers.

Pages 284, 285, 287: The answers are listed in alphabetical order.

dream   help   honest   joyful   search   verb

Page 286: The answers for this page are listed in the correct order.

I and A	last row	last column
T and Y	R	second row and fourth column

First answer: The top line should read **2, 6, 3, 4, 1, 5**

Clues: First, fill in all rows and columns that are only missing one number or letter.

Page 288

Grid one: The bottom line is missing **1**. The first column on the left is missing **4**, then **6**.

Grid two: The top row is missing **61**. The last column on the right is missing **57**, then **59**, then **62**.

Page 289

Grid one: The first row is missing **B**, then **A**. The first column is missing **A**.

Grid two: The fifth row is missing **P**. The fifth column is missing **0**.

First answer: (#1 on Oak to #2 on Long).

Take Oak south to Tuller. Take Tuller west to Long. Take Long south to #2.

Other longer routes are also possible.

Clues: Lightly circle in pencil the two places you are going between. Write your answer and refer to the map, then erase your pencil marks. You could use a colored marker on the map to show the routes you would take between the two places.

Pages 292, 293, 294: Map Reading

First answer: Parking Lot 4

Clues: Some questions may have more than one possible answer. Lightly mark the starting point and read the question. Write your answer on the lines as you refer to the map or use a colored pencil or marker to show the answer on the map.

Pages 295, 296: Map Construction

First answer: Troy

Clues: The first letter of each street is listed in order.

2. C	3. L	4. R	5. F	6. M	7. W	8. H
9. P	10. S	11. S	12. L	13. N	14. V	15. B
16. K	17. G	18. D	19. O	20. W		

Pages 297, 298: Map Locations

First answer: 14

Clues: The answers are identified by the boxed number. The answer boxes are listed in chronological order. Only seventeen of the numbered boxes are used as answers.

1   5   9   10   12   19   21   25   26   32   36   38   39   41   42   50

Pages 299, 300: Codes

First answer: The first two words in code 1 are: My doctor

Clues: The first two words are listed.

Code 2: The mail   Code 3: Definition of

Pages 301, 302, 303, 304, 305: Project Planning

First Answer: The first clue tells you to write blouses in the bottom box on the left and jackets in the bottom box on the right. The second clue tells you that scarves are in a top box and in the middle of the closet. Write scarves into the third box across on top.

Clues: One of the answers for each problem is listed.

Page 302: The pasta is on the top shelf on the left and the spices are directly below.

Page 303: Place Penney's and Macy's in two corners across from each other diagonally and place Dimensions and Gap on the other corners.

Page 304: The top row in order is: pumpkins, pumpkins, and tomatoes.

Page 305: Add to your information that Jeff and Robert are Christopher's sons.

Pages 306, 307, 308, 309: Schedule Planning

First Answer: The first thing on Mary's schedule is to go to the post office at 9am. The clue for this is the sentence: "There is usually a line at the post office by 9:30, so . . . Mary likes to go there before then."

Clues: A random answer from each schedule is listed.

Page 306: At 11:30 Mary goes to the shoe repair shop.

Page 307: The seventh stop on the tour is Fifth Avenue.

Page 308: Act 5 is really Intermission.

Page 309: The desk will be taken off at stop 7.

Pages 310, 311, 312, 313, 314: Logic Problems

First Answer: Amy, on the top line, has the cocker.

Clues: The answer having to do with the first person is listed for each item. Circle that answer in the row next to the person's name. Cross off that possible answer from the rest of the columns.

Page 311: Barb is the banker.   Chris is 50 years old.

Page 312: The Bakers are going to Chicago.   Megan had steak for dinner.

Page 313: Anna and Tom are married.   The Howes live in a tan house.

Page 314: Bud lives in Miami.   Jean's last name is Johnson.

Pages 315, 316, 317, 318, 319, 320, 321, 322: Situational Logic

First Answer: The answer is the third choice. It makes sense that a boy in third grade is not tall enough to hit all the buttons that go from 1 on the bottom to 10 at the top. It is easy for him to hit the button to the first floor on the way to school, but he is too short to reach up to the 10th button.

Clues: You can eliminate one of the choices from all of the questions. The first choice is always wrong. Cross out all of the first answers and choose from the second or third answer.

Pages 323, 324, 325, 326, 327, 328, 329, 330: Literal Meaning, Tricky Questions

First Answer: Page 323 – It is the same distance. An hour and a half is the same as 90 minutes.

Page 327 – The president would still be the president even if the vice-president died.

Clues: A clue, an answer, or short hint is listed for each situation. The hints are in scrambled order.

daughter	it won't lay	Mary	triplets	5 more
1, 2, 3, 4	throw it up	win	charcoal	letter **M**
spare tire	played other people	lions	94 pounds	all 26
your name	12 stamps	drive-in	5 children	none
Everest	fictional characters	elevator	nowhere	2 ears
yesterday . . .	owes 10	women	deaf	bald
more wishes	every year	remove **S**	corn on the cob	
2 errors	natural causes	10 minutes		